Chakras
and
Chakra Healing
for Beginners

A BEGINNERS GUIDE TO THE CHAKRAS - LEARN ALL ABOUT CHAKRA BALANCING, CHAKRA AWAKENING AND SELF-HEALING

Aurora White

Copyright (c) Aurora White

Thank you for getting our book!

If you enjoy using it and you found it useful in your journey of spiritual growth and healing, we would greatly appreciate your review on Amazon.

Just head on over to this book's Amazon page and click "Write a customer review".

We read each and every one of them. Thanks!

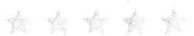

Contents

Introduction 7

Chapter 1: Getting to Know the Chakra System 11
- Indian roots 11
- Chakras and Buddhism 13
- Chakras 14
- Chakras and deities 16
- How it was practiced 18
- What is a balanced chakra? 19
- Chakras and the west 20

Chapter 2: Connection between Human Life and Energies of the Body 23
- Benjamin's biotic energy theory 23
- Alternate theories of human life and energy 25
  - 1.1 Plato's theory of the soul 25
  - 1.2 Human biofield, local field, and meridians 26
  - 1.3 The theory behind Reiki 27
  - 1.4 Everything is energy: Basics of quantum physics and the chakra system 29
- Methods of alternate healthcare derived from energy theories 30
- Is alternate medicine evidence based? 30
- A word from alternative medicine practitioners 31
- The future of energy medicine 33

Chapter 3: Chakras Explained by Science 34
- What does psychology say about the chakra system? 35

    1.1 Cognitive psychology and chakras ...35
    1.2 Anodea Judith and Maslow's
         hierarchy of needs 36
    1.3 Erikson's theory and chakras.............37
Scientific evidence for the
basis of the chakra system.......................... 38
    1.4 Wisneski and Anderson's application
         of integrative medicine 39
    1.5 The pineal gland 40
    1.6 Mind and body experiment by
         Dr. Dispenza 41
    1.7 The endocrine system and chakras 42

Chapter 4: The Root Chakra 45

Location of the root chakra 46
Significance of the root chakra 47
General features of the root chakra................47
An unbalanced root chakra.............................. 50
Signs of unbalanced root chakra 50
Root chakra healing meditation 53
    1.1 Affirmation mantra.............................53
    1.2 Yoga Asana...54
    1.3 Aromatherapy....................................54
    1.4 Crystal therapy 55
    1.5 Sound therapy....................................55
Root Chakra Guided Meditation
    Bringing balance to the root chakra 55
Meditation guide... 56
    Beginning the session:................................ 56

Chapter 5: The Sacral Chakra 59

Facts about the sacral chakra 60
Unbalanced sacral chakra signs...................... 62
Sacral chakra meditation techniques 64
Sacral chakra guided meditation.................... 66
    Meditation guide: 67

Meditation script 67

Chapter 6: Solar Plexus Chakra 69

Functions of the solar plexus chakra 70
Symptoms of unbalanced solar plexus
    chakra 71
Meditation techniques 73
Solar plexus chakra meditation script 74

Chapter 7: The Heart Chakra 79

Functions of heart chakra 80
How to spot an unbalanced heart chakra 82
Therapeutic remedies for heart chakra 85
Meditation guide 88

Chapter 8: The Throat Chakra 91

Significance of throat chakra 91
Unbalanced throat chakra symptoms 94
Throat chakra meditation techniques 96
Meditation guide for throat chakra 100

Chapter 9: The Third Eye Chakra 103

What makes the third eye chakra
    important? 104
What are the symptoms of an
    unbalanced third eye chakra? 106
How to open your third eye chakra
    at home 109
Third eye chakra guided meditation 112

Chapter 10: The Crown Chakra 115

How an open crown chakra functions 116
Signs your crown chakra is imbalanced 118
How to heal your crown chakra 121
Meditation guide for crown chakra 124
Final Thoughts 126
Endnotes 129

INTRODUCTION

Does the image of a torso silhouette with different colored lights on various focal points ring any bells for you? It's very likely that you've come across this several times in your life. Often individuals find it appealing to the eye, but the meaning behind this imagery is more than just the aesthetics. Such drawings that you come across are actually referring to the age-old concept of chakras. Upon hearing this terminology, many individuals get intrigued, but confusion can easily arise. While it is easy to observe the human body through the skin, bone, and muscle structure, what is complicated about chakras is their invisibility to the naked eye[1]. Chakras are intangible and require a bit more sensitivity to get noticed. However, once you begin working on your chakras, it can help you bring positive change in your life through a strong connection between your mind, body, and soul.

Often individuals question what exactly chakras are. Pronounced as **cha**·kruh, this terminology is borrowed from Sanskrit. The word can loosely be translated as 'wheel'. However, the essential reference for this word is the 'wheel of life[2]'. This analogy comes from the delicate anatomy that governs the flow of life and energy through our bodily structures. These energy hubs in our body are responsible for our physiological, psychological, and emotional health. It is vital for our well-being that the flow of life is smooth and without any flaw.

When the current of energy flowing through your chakras is interrupted either completely or partially, the symptoms of this blockage appear on three levels. These points include your body, mind, and soul. Nevertheless, getting to know your chakras and working on their health can bring the tranquility in your life that all human beings aim to achieve. To ponder on this further, we can refer to a personal journey of an individual who overcame the troubles of life by getting in touch with his chakras. John Graybill II attempted to work on his chakras to get back control of his life and his happiness. Starting his journey in 2010, he saw his life shifting the day he began doing yoga with Master Han. Through his discovery of chakras, he was able to cultivate a deeper understanding of energy, spirituality, and the power one has within[3].

Drawing from such personal experiences of other people, you might have felt inspired to begin your own journey of healing as well. In case Western medicine has not proven to be effective for your medical conditions, know that there is an alternative. Chakra healing is such a substitute that can help you resolve any underlying set of troubles that could be making your body hard to function and overflowing your daily life with stress and other mental health difficulties.

In this book, you will find everything that a beginner needs to know about chakra healing. While most people want to jump on this and begin their therapeutic journey right away, it has been noted that this process is, in fact, a life-long journey with lasting effects that will stay with you for the rest of your days once you get into learning all about chakras. As with any other subject, to understand chakras best, it is essential to observe where they come from, their roots, significance, benefits, and finally, how to make them healthy[4].

CHAPTER 1

Getting to Know the Chakra System

Chakra is a word you must have already heard while mingling with your friends or during your yoga classes. However, do you really know what it means? If the answer is a hard no, the good thing is that you are not alone in this journey. You might know what chakra is in a broader sense but the understanding of this Sanskrit term is beyond a single word translation. You must be eager to just begin with your chakra journey but word of the wise is to invest some time in knowing the history behind this age-old concept and practice. When you will get to know the chakra system with us, you will not just become the master of this technique but you will be able to build a deep connection with it.

INDIAN ROOTS

As mentioned earlier, chakras are a number of energy centers of our body. The concept of chakras is a prehistoric one. This practice comes from Hinduism and it also has its roots in Buddhism which will be discussed in the next section. These central points of our body are in charge of our psychic and bodily functions. They merge and interact with each other in order to communicate and make sure we are functioning at our optimum level. Going back in history, the theory of chakra is derived from an ancient text called the Vedas. Additional framework of the chakra system includes Shri Jabala Darshana Upanishad, the Yoga-Shikka Upanishad, the Cudamini Upanishad and the Shandilya Upanishad[5]. All of these scriptures give information about the location of chakras and their symbolic descriptions. Though, in the tenth century Guru Goraknath wrote his version of the chakra system known as 'Gorakshashatakam'. Widely known as a saint of his time, his text provided his disciples with new knowledge regarding the chakra practice. He was the person who established a connection between awakening the chakra and use of meditation as a technique to do that[6]. It was only in 1918 that this scripture was translated into English. This indicates that while in the West the practice of chakra healing was introduced approximately 100 years ago, it has existed for centuries in the subcontinent.

In the original text, the authors maintain that the purpose of the chakra system is to function as a model for *nyasa*[7]. The latter term means that in ancient times the chakra system was practiced in order to install the deity-energies at specific spots on the human body. There are several outstanding features of the chakra system that the original sources highlight. The first key feature of chakras is that each of them is associated with a specific element such as water, fire, wind, space and earth. The next point to note about the chakra system is that each chakra is also linked to a specific Hindu deity. The authors of this system also suggest that this practice is culture-specific. Yogis have believed that the sound of Sanskrit language makes unique and powerful vibrations that brings spiritual liberation to our chakras. That is why chanting in Sanskrit was practiced during chakra meditation.

Chakras and Buddhism

The lineage of chakras can also be traced in Tibetan Buddhism. Known as channel wheels, this concept utilized the mapping of chakras. In Buddhism, this terminology is used in a slightly difference sense and it denotes that concept of rebirth. The Tibetan Buddhism is a surviving branch of the Indian Vajrayana. This school of belief is mainly influenced by yoga practices. It is mostly found in Nepal, Mongolia, Bhutan and Tibet. According to this branch of Buddhism the chakras play a key role in attaining Buddhahood. The chakras are opened in stages and an attempt is made to bring all the energy to the central channel of the body to meet this target. This way the Tibetan Buddhists used to obtain a clear conscience and look at the word beyond its material worth. Although it should be noted that in most

Tibetan Buddhist schools, the knowledge of chakras is passed from a teacher to a student. This means that it is rarely shared outside this formal dynamic of teaching[8].

In addition to this, the Chinese Mahayana Buddhists often teach the chakra system in combination with Qi-Gong, Tai-Chi and other forms of energy control and management. These exercises, similar to the chakra system, focus on developing an individual's psychosomatic abilities. At least three of the seven main chakras are recognized by this branch of Buddhism. These chakras include the ones located at the lower abdomen, head, and chest.

Chakras

In Sanskrit the continuous energy flow through the chakra system is called 'shakti'. The basic understanding of the chakras is that all of the seven chakras are aligned with our spine. That means that each chakra is also linked with various parts of the human nerve system, the organs and the glands. Numerous early texts note down more than the seven popular chakras but as the concept has refined over the years, the focus is only maintained on a handful of chakras[9].

- **Sahasrara** also known as the *Crown Chakra*: This energy channel is placed on the highest level of the body; the head. Yogis believe that through this chakra humans build a connection with the divine.

- **Ajna** also known as the *Third Eye Chakra*: On the second level of our body, this chakra is placed on our forehead right between the eyes. This energy channel is linked to our sense of purpose in life, finding the direction of our life and our intuition.

- **Vishuddha** also known as the *Throat Chakra*: Coming to the third level of our body, this energy vortex is found near the throat. Across all the ancient texts, this chakra is held responsible for our sense of self expression.

- **Anahata** also known as the *Heart Chakra*: This chakra is located near our heart. A good energy flow through the heart chakra helps us take control of love and relationships. Additionally, it also controls our ability of self-acceptance. Most people like to mention that the heart chakra is the hub of human emotions.

- **Manipura** also known as the *Solar Plexus Chakra*: Slightly lower than the heart, this chakra is placed somewhere around our abdomen. Due to its location, this chakra is mainly concerned with maintaining balance and power on ourselves.

- **Swadhisthana** also known as the *Sacral Chakra*: This chakra is mainly located near our lower abdomen. Concerned with our reproductive system, the sacral chakra is in charge of our sexual health, sexual emotions, and pleasure. Some sources mention that the exact location of this channel is 2 inches below the navel.

- **Muladhara** also known as *Root Chakra*: This is the lowest stage of the chakra system and the energy recycling is mainly concerned with the root chakra. Opening the human kundalini means mastering the technique of meditation so that there is a healthy energy flow through our root chakra. Once that happens, we are able to feel whole. That means that we attain a sense of belonging and achieve high-grade success in our career.

CHAKRAS AND DEITIES

As mentioned earlier, each energy channel is linked to a Hindu god or goddess. The specific characteristics of these deities can tell you more about each chakra. In olden times, the ritual of opening chakras and attaining a healthy energy flow was to satisfy these deities and obtain their magical powers. Usually when you are taught about the chakra system this detail is often overlooked. Nevertheless, a brief note on this superficial link between chakras and these deities will spark further interest in you to begin your chakra expedition[10].

- The **Crown Chakra** is believed to be linked with the Hindu deity *Shiva*. Also known as 'The Father' this Hindu god holds the role of transformer and destroyer. Through him the crown chakra is rebalanced and humans gain his qualities of will, purpose and power.

- The **Third Eye Chakra** is allegedly controlled by two deities which include *Vishnu* and *Krishna*. Linked with the element of soul also called *Atma* in Sanskrit, these two gods are saviors and sustainers. Through meditation, humans can open this specific chakras and gain the qualities of love and wisdom.

- The **Throat Chakra** is associated with the Hindu goddess *Saraswati*. It is also ruled by *Brahma* who is popularly known as the Holy Spirit. These two deities are linked to the element of space. Ancient yogis believed that those blessed with a healthy throat chakra can experience creative and active intelligence.

- The **Heart Chakra** is controlled by lord *Hanuman* as well as previously mentioned *Brahma*. These two deities belong to the element of air and therefore their power

- The **Solar Plexus Chakra** is the territory of *Laxmi*. Belonging to the element of fire, this goddess is denoted by her qualities of abundance and prosperity. That is why those who open their solar plexus chakra experience the ability to develop concrete knowledge.

- The **Sacral Chakra** is controlled by goddess *Parvati* and the Holy Spirit *Brahma*. Both of these deities control the element of water. Their power gives them the abilities of passion and self-sacrifice. That is why people who have a healthy sacral chakra are believed to be extremely devoted beings.

- The **Root Chakra** is located at the lower part of our body which is why it is linked with the element of Earth. With that, lord *Ganesha* and *Brahma* are the two gods who fuel this chakra with their power and bring order to our chaotic mind, body and soul[11].

How it was practiced

Throughout history, there were several methods used by different schools of chakra system to get in tune with the human body and maintain this internal energy system. Yet, measuring out whether one is making progress or not has always been a hard task. The obvious reason behind this difficulty is the unseen nature of these chakras. Although, the disciples of yogis mentioned being able to feel their chakras as they practiced olden techniques to open these energy channels.

One of the most commonly known ritual related to the chakra system is called *chakra bathing*. True to its name, this technique was believed to help cleanse the stagnant energies of the chakra system and keep each of the wheel open at all times. Similar to our mind and bodily functions, yogis believed that something could accumulate these invisible channels and block their strength. Chakra bathing was practiced by choosing the chakra one wants to open in step one[12]. After that, a sacred space was needed to run a bath preferably in a clean tub. Dim light usually helped in building concentration. After that, adding healing elements such as oils, herbs and crystals connected to the specific chakra was suggested. Lastly, yogis kept a relaxed state of mind and began to meditate in order to activate their chakras.

What is a balanced chakra?

A large part of the chakra system and getting to know it is understanding what chakra balancing stands for. There are three main states of our chakra system;

blocked chakra, imbalanced chakra and balanced chakra. All the knowledge that you will gather about the chakra system is extremely valuable for effectively balancing your chakra. This is our end goal; to be able to balance your chakra. A balanced chakra is one where the energy flow is smooth and without any interruption.

If the chakra is imbalanced that can mean two things; either the energy flowing through your wheel of life is very little or most of the energy is only flowing through a few of the chakras causing these precise energy vortexes to be heavily charged. A blocked chakra occurs when there is no energy flowing through these energy centers. That also means that there is no communication between them and so this state, if prolonged, can become a cause of severe human body and mind conditions. The goal of learning about the chakra system is simple; it is to avoid these states of chakras and make sure you restore equilibrium in your chakra system[13].

CHAKRAS AND THE WEST

The number of ancient sources that exist about the chakra system are very confusing when compared with each other. Collectively, the scripture and schools of the chakra system denote different key characteristics of each chakra. With that, the number of existing chakras has always been a subject for debate. It is surprising to notice that even after a chaotic historical background, this ancient practice was able to make its way to the West.

According to numerous analyzers, the chakra system was able to come to the West through a Sanskrit text written by Punananda Yati back in 1577. Other than that, a 13th century scripture called 'Sarasvati's Ornament' also contributes to the Western understanding of the chakra system. Although a simple problem that lies within these two texts was the number of chakras they recognize. When the chakra system was adapted by the West, most Indian yogis who passed this ancient knowledge to the West recognized only seven main chakras from Punananda's book. The translation of this book was done by John Woodroffe in 1918 and that is when chakra healing made its entrance in the West. While this translation was very complicated, other books were written by Anodea Judith such as 'Eastern Body, Western Mind' is one of the most followed scriptures in the West[14].

The American hippie culture is also credited for bringing and popularizing this Indian practice to the West[15]. In the early 90s, people belonging to this subgroup travelled to India and became disciples of various tantric yogis. After being thoroughly trained by them, they brought the chakra system with them and began teaching the West about it. While the popularity of the chakra system was low in early years, today it has become one of the focal points of the

Western society. You can find numerous companies selling healing oils, crystals and guidance books about the chakra system. However, there is a huge difference between the Western model of the chakra system and the Indian model of chakra structure. While the Hindu model of this system is quite complex, the Western adaptation of the chakra system is much more global because of its easy understanding and limited vocabulary.

CHAPTER 2

Connection between Human Life and Energies of the Body

How did life begin on Earth? While this is a bigger question, the expected answer is always a simple one. Still, the various schools of human life make it a difficult concept to understand. What is intriguing about human lifecycle is that our existence did not immediately start right after the Earth was made. Instead, we began habituating the world millions of years later. Throughout human history, we have believed that everyone exists because we are the creation of a higher being. Various religions tackle this notion in different ways and generate a contradictory view point of life on Earth and the human body itself. However, while a belief system helps us understand the purpose we must have as humans, to comprehend how human life continues to exist requires a much detailed analysis of theories coming from various cultures, prehistoric times, religions as well as objective science itself.

BENJAMIN'S BIOTIC ENERGY THEORY

Since the 19th century objective science has believed that the human body just like all living things is made up of cells which come in different shapes and sizes. Firstly discovered in 17th century, modern microscopes of that period revealed the difference between cells found in many species of living things. What gives various species life was explained and concluded on the basis of this observation. However, there were two other theories that suggested human life is different than other living organisms. These theories were a mixture of religious guidelines and scientific research.

By early 1800s, scientists discovered some substances that made human life unique. One chemical that was observed in humans was called urea. Excreted through urine, this chemical gave life to the theory of vitalism. It was believed that only living things develop such chemicals and scientists went on to suggest that these chemicals are infused with life energy. However, because a German chemist was able to make this chemical outside of the human body and this theory lost its popularity right away[16].

Nevertheless, the extension of vitalism was brought by Benjamin Moore. The biochemist studied molecular physics for numerous years as well as the structure of living organisms. He rejected all material based explanations of living organisms but he also opposed any spiritual explanations of human life. Instead, he introduced the concept of 'biotic theory' through his book called 'The Origin and Nature of Life'. Through this theory, Benjamin claimed that there was a presence of energy in all living bodies that cannot be explained or measured using basic physics and chemistry principles[17]. Although, because his theory could not be proven using the fundamentals of scientific research, it was quickly rejected. His theory was only carried forward by a few of his disciples but in mainstream science it is overlooked till today due to lack of palpable evidence.

ALTERNATE THEORIES OF HUMAN LIFE AND ENERGY

1.1 Plato's theory of the soul

When it comes to building a connection between human life and energies of the body, scientific theories are not the best at giving an explanation because they are based on the principles of measurable and tangible proof. What gives life to alternate medicine such as energy healing are theories developed based on philosophy and intuition. One such theory of life was written by Plato. A revolutionist and extremely advanced Greek philosopher, Plato had different views about the existence of life.

Plato believed that the human existence on earth is a small shadow of a higher spiritual plane and the physical body is a mere vessel that traps the soul and restricts it from reaching that spiritual plane. He also suggested that the vessel is capable of death but the soul, which gives the human body energy to function, continues to live on. As a dualist, he also believed that humans are dual creatures; the first part is the human body and the second part is the energies found in the body. He further suggested that the soul is immortal and continues to live on but the human body is dependent on the existence of energy in order to survive[18]. Although Plato's work is completely rejected by researchers, it gives way to various healing techniques that are guaranteed to work for mainstream population.

1.2 Human biofield, local field, and meridians

One pillar of energy medicine is the theory that there are several energy fields that work together to govern all fundamental biological processes. There are three types of energy fields that are responsible for the functions of all living things. The first is called *biofield*. This energy field is located around the body and it was also measured scientifically because of its electromagnetic properties that were easily revealed by Burr's laboratory. In alternate medicine, this type of energy is commonly known as the 'aura' of a living thing. Those who tested this energy field suggested that *biofield* has the capability to hold information about a specific organism and transmit that information throughout that organism.

The second type of energy field is called the *local field*. Contrary to the principles of *biofield*, the *local field* is concerned with certain parts of the body. Similar to the chakra system, the energy here is concentrated in particular areas of an organism such as the organs and so on. What is interesting about the *local field* is that it was measured scientifically by Valarie Hunt. This UCLA researcher demonstrated specific regions of the human skin that produced rapid electrical oscillations. Although her study has not gained popularity in the scientific world, it supports the existence of the chakra system. These vortexes of biophysical energy are dependent on the external and internal energy fields[19].

Lastly, the third part of this energy system is concerned with the regulation of energies within a living organism and is widely known as 'energy pathways'. In traditional Chinese context, these pathways are known as meridians. A study was conducted in 1998 with the use of fMRI (functional Magnetic Resonance Imaging) and acupuncture technique[20]. Stimulating an acupuncture area in the toe seemed to have activated the exact areas of the brain that were predicted by this ancient acupuncture theory without any prior research back in the days. This suggested that the meridian system operates similar to a field that is independent of our physical body and is concerned more with the energies accumulating our body. Moreover, that means that our body functions cannot be carried out without the presence of this invisible energy pathway.

1.3 The theory behind Reiki

Reiki is an age-old healing practice that started during prehistoric times and it has now become a major part of the contemporary world. While Reiki is formally known as a therapy technique, there is an interesting theory behind it. Reiki is a combination of Japanese and Chinese words where 'rei' stands for spiritual and 'ki' means vital energy. One of the key ideas of this technique is that there is vital energy that is channeled through the body and it provides essential support to the body's ability to heal itself naturally. Yet because of no scientific evidence to support the claim of vital energy, the NCCIH does not recognize Reiki as a useful form of health-related therapy. Despite the fact that Reiki lacks a scientific backbone, it has become part of various health care organizations including state hospitals.

The origins of Reiki are spiritual in nature. It dates back to 19th century and it is linked to a popular Japanese monk named Mikao Usui[21]. He drew his healing techniques from philosophies of traditional Asian practices. The root of this methodology is the belief that imbalances in our body's vital energy are the cause of physical disease. Correcting this imbalance promotes healthy and healed human bodies. By 1937, Hawayo Takata brought this method to the West and since then it has been extremely common in Western medical practices.

Another basis of the Reiki therapy is borrowed from the previously mentioned biofield theory. However, unlike other alternate energy healing practices, Reiki is slightly different. Instead of focusing on rearranging the body's biofield, Reiki works passively. Reiki can be extremely soothing and the results are often quickly displayed because the Reiki healer is only concerned with balancing the biofield of our body instead of completely changing its state.

1.4 Everything is energy: Basics of quantum physics and the chakra system

Because Quantum physics is a widely accepted theory, this branch of science can be used to prove the existence of the chakra system. According to this school of physics, everything is made of energy. Their research has also proven this fact. The common factor between Quantum physics and spirituality is that they both connect with the ideology that energy is central to every living organism and forms the core of living bodies[22]. Although, Quantum physics also suggests that even inanimate object is made of energy which is where it differentiates from the chakra system. As the movement of energy is essential for life, how we think, function and breathe is dependent on the electrical energy that is flowing through our body. Even while resting, this energy is responsible for our state of mind and body.

However, because Quantum physics is not magic, the claim that the chakra system is deeply rooted with the ancient deities as mentioned earlier cannot be supported. Still, when applied to the human body, many believe that Quantum physics has made claims that go hand in hand with ancient theories about the connection between human body and energy[23].

Methods of alternate healthcare derived from energy theories

In order to grasp a better understanding of the connection between human life and energy theories, exploring how these concepts are applied to alternate healthcare is mandatory. Have you heard about any energy healthcare methods? The chances are that you have informally come across them but usually you are recommended to follow Western medicine. That is because Western medicine is not only backed up by scientific research but it is also a major opponent of alternate methods. However, these alternate energy healing techniques have been practiced by us for centuries today.

Is alternate medicine evidence based?

Complementary healthcare is a group of different medical care systems, practices, and theories that at present are not considered as part of conventional health care practice. Nonetheless, over the years the list of complementary medical practice has increased. Ayurveda is one such alternative health care system which comes from India and has existed for approximately 5,000 years now. To briefly describe this technique, Ayurveda is a combination of herbs, massages, meditation, and yoga. All of these methodologies come from the previously mentioned theories regarding energy healing.

While there is a lack of evidence that shows any correlation between energy healing techniques and good health, the use of such techniques has been increasing. In 1998, it was noticed that 42.1% Americans were using complementary therapies. By 2002, out of the 45.2% patients at least 11.6% were practicing breathing meditation while the rest made yoga and body work daily part of their lives[24]. The increasing number of complementary medicine use and the fact that individuals are able to make it part of their routine serves as a fact that there must be some truth to the idea that human life is a consequence of energy channels located in our bodies.

A WORD FROM ALTERNATIVE MEDICINE PRACTITIONERS

Yogis have had the chance to learn what energy healing is about throughout their lives. Not only do they have access to detailed knowledge about the subject but they also have the experience to validate their belief. With that, they interact with numerous disciples and patients and they are able to notice the beneficial effects of what they are practicing through the individuals they treat.

According to alternate medicine practitioners the human body is only able to operate in harmony because of the energy system which is derived from the universe around us. The empty space that we can often observe holds latticework of various energies which vibrate at different frequencies. These vibrations from the space around us encompass our mental, physical, spiritual, and emotional features. Yogis believe that the human body has the ability to heal itself and return to its natural state[25]. While most critics call this belief supernatural with no grounding, yogis think that reconnecting with ancient Indian wisdom is the best way for self-healing. After all, our ancestors were able to find the right balance through this knowledge and in that time there was no concept of quantitative research.

This universal life force flows through all living beings and help us gain back our ability to self-heal in case it has been interrupted due to poor diet, mental health, and environmental conditions. However, the therapies that are derived from belief in energy channels are majorly dependent on two things; client's ability to maintain a clear and conscious mind and the healer's intervention and skills[26]. That is why unlike Western medicine, each patient is unique and a tailored energy healing regimen works for them but not for someone else. Overall, healers do acknowledge that because the next generation is born during modern age, understanding the complex nature of this belief system is often tough. Though, the best possible way to find a connection between human life and universal energy is seeing it for yourself.

THE FUTURE OF ENERGY MEDICINE

What lies in the future for these theories and therapies is vastly dependent upon the flexibility of Western medicine. Currently the mainstream medical model depends on the mixture of basic principles of physics and biochemistry. While physics is used to diagnose any underlying health condition, biochemistry model is used to treat it effectively. However, accepting that the human life is dependent upon energy fields and cellular and molecular communication system is outside the central ideology of Western medicine. Nevertheless, the future perspective regarding alternate medicine includes bridging the gap between allopathic therapies and energy medicine in such a way that it is deeply cohesive. For example, accepting the possibility that the endocrine system and the chakra system overlap gives a complex answer to this medical debate[27]. Not only does it add to the explanation of an underlying disease but it also comes in handy by increasing the number of treatments available to tackle a problem. With that, the probability of a patient getting better also heightens.

CHAPTER 3

Chakras Explained by Science

The chakra system is a basic concept of how the human body functions but it is often overlooked by scientific research. One probable cause of scientific withdrawal is the description of chakras. For objective scientists, chakras have always been a part of ancient mythology and ideology that is not quantifiable. As a result, no explanation regarding the influence of chakras on our physiological function has been broadly recognized by scientists as well as a handful of yoga scholars. The main problem behind this obstacle is recognizing chakra and yoga as a subjective experience. That is why other than the scientists, some authors of the chakra system avoid replacing subjective explanations with objective ones[28]. This takes us back to a popular debate between positivists and other schools of thought. The application of uniform measuring tools on subjective matters is nearly impossible because such level of control cannot be practiced on matters that are highly complex and involve human experiences. Though, as the debate about any correlation between science and chakras continues there are various explanations that are often applied to this energy medicine technique.

WHAT DOES PSYCHOLOGY SAY ABOUT THE CHAKRA SYSTEM?

Psychologists recognize that believers of the chakra system are more prone to experiencing physical, mental, and emotional effects of this practice. While yoga scholars use terminologies like 'nerve centers' and 'sites of major organ' to support the existence of energy channels, cognitive psychology has a different view regarding this matter. Using the principles of objective science, cognitive psychology studies the mind and backs its theories through scientific and tangible evidence only. According to this school, the proposal that our body structure includes metaphysical centers cannot be supported by modern scientific explanations.

1.1 Cognitive psychology and chakras

Cognitive psychology has its own theory regarding practices like yoga, chakra meditation, and crystal healing. Under the lenses of this school of thought, one main cognitive aspect that most likely contributes to the effects of chakra meditation is confirmation bias. As many individuals claim that they are able to experience the promised changes of chakra healing, the reason behind that is remembering the times when improvements occurred in their well-being just after they started believing in the chakra system. In other words, our mind tricks us to believe that we are getting better. The healing might just be because of external factors such as taking medication, improved diet, a healthy fitness routine and so on[29].

In addition to this, there are social factors that are more likely to influence our belief in the chakra system. The chakra system comes from a collectivist society where a strict relation is made between the elders and the young. Often termed as authority bias, psychologists believe that in such cultures the tendency of accepting the opinion of an authority figure is more likely to occur. Even in the West, because leaders of yoga practice often have more experience, new disciples become more prone to accepting them as authority figures and hence believing in the existence of what they teach. That is how psychology believes that the chakra system is unfit for scientific understanding and does not use it to explain how the human body functions.

1.2 Anodea Judith and Maslow's hierarchy of needs

The Maslow's hierarchy of needs is an outline of requirements that one must satisfy for growth. These needs should be satisfied in an orderly fashion so that individuals can move to the next level of the hierarchy. Adonea Judith in her book 'Eastern Body, Western Mind: Psychology and the Chakra System as a Path to the Self' compares this energy medicine theory with Maslow's model of needs.

According to Judith, Maslow's need for medical safety is compared with the root chakra. She associates the need for safety with the sacral chakra and sense of belonging with the solar plexus chakra. Judith goes on to compare the need for healthy self-esteem with the heart chakra and state of self-actualization with the throat chakra. Lastly, she mentions that the state of transcendence in Maslow's hierarchy is linked with the crown chakra and the third eye chakra. In this manner, Judith suggests that each of these chakras are a representation of human needs that must be met in order to guarantee survival and progress[30].

1.3 Erikson's theory and chakras

Anodea Judith also took a look at other Western paradigms related to psychology. She particularly analyzed Erikson's stages of psychosocial development and suggested it overlaps with the chakra system. This model suggests that human personality develops in a prearranged manner from infancy to adult life. Judith especially picked out the 'trust vs. mistrust' stage of development to compare with root and sacral energy vortexes. With this comparison, Judith says that our root and sacral chakras are responsible for human development. She maintains that if these chakras are not healthy, humans develop mistrust in their life. However, if these chakras are healthy, the opposite can take place[31].

In general, Judith understood that there indeed is a lack of empirical research that can prove or disapprove the existence of chakra system. In that case, while medical science cannot develop factual basis of this ancient theory, there are a lot of psychological models that can be useful for the chakra system in order to give it a backbone. Still, while these psychological applications do help us understand the chakra system better they still lack evidence based research. Although, it can be debated that just like the chakra system, many of these psychology models were created without empirical data but their application to real life problems has proven to show positive results.

Scientific Evidence for the Basis of the Chakra System

Those who believe there is science behind the chakra system apply various scientific studies and explanations on this prehistoric energy medicine technique. Empirical studies have shown that mental states such as stress and relaxation can affect our physical state. When our body is under stress it releases powerful hormones that generate anxiety. Just like that, stress can become a contributing factor to developing serious physical illnesses as recognized by the National Institute of Health. According to this theory, our mental health has a direct relation with our physical health.

The knowledge behind this claim comes from Robert Ader's experiment which was conducted in 1975. This researcher was able to provide palpable evidence that our thoughts can alter our immune system. He was inspired by a previous researcher known as William Osler. Through Osler's experiment it was noticed that an asthma patient was asked to smell an artificial rose without any prior knowledge regarding the nature of the object. This resulted in a physiological response; an asthma attack. Ader drew several conclusions from his research. He suggested that mammals are capable of conditioning their immune system and response[32]. Connecting this theory with chakras and Eastern medicine, the claim that energy flows through our bodies and produces biological alterations can be demonstrated. Ader's research led many individuals to contradict the previously mentioned cognitive psychology application of the chakra system. He was able to showcase that it is not that our mind is tricking us to believe that chakra healing is in the works but that our mind has the ability to negatively and positively impact our immune system.

1.4 Wisneski and Anderson's application of integrative medicine

These two authors wrote a popular book known as 'The Scientific Basis of Integrative Medicine' back in 2005 which is often used to provide support energy medicine. With over 20 years of research, the authors were able to compile several pieces of evidence that supports energy medicine. Wisneski and Anderson note down the theta healing system that can explain the physiological benefits of deep relaxation which is a major part of meditation. Research shows that the alpha and theta state of mind can release certain relaxation hormones that result in substantial benefit in terms of our emotional and physical health. These include melatonin, anandamide, benzodiazepines, and other chemicals already present in the human body. The existence of such hormones which are triggered by a relaxed mind provide biological strength to Eastern medicine. They also add that in order to activate this physiological healing system a connection between the mind and body is required[33].

1.5 The pineal gland

The pineal gland in our body is responsible for linking the external environment with our internal body systems. This gland takes external information and converts it into a chemical and/or electrical signals to send it to our organs. The pineal gland converts temperature, light, and magnetic rays present in the environment and turns them into neuroendocrine signals which are responsible for regulating the human body. With that the research has also shows that it can regulate our internal clock which determines when we go to sleep and when we wake up. Such in depth studies conducted over the period of 30 years claim that in this case it is not the pituitary gland but the pineal gland that is the master of our endocrine system.

Taking from this establishment, Wisneski and Anderson correlate the pineal gland with the mythical third eye chakra as well as the ideology of sixth sense. They maintain that this ancient wisdom might be the physiological interface that connects the mind and body. The pineal gland can be looked at as a gatekeeper between our experiences that excel the five senses. The researchers further theorize that the pineal gland might be the physiological channel that interfaces with these ancient energy portals from Eastern medicine[34]. The reason behind that is the basic role of this gland. It is an energy transducer that sends hormonal and electrical message through our body which is exactly what the chakra system is about. Various forms of energy such as sound, light, and electromagnetism are translated into electrical and chemical signals that flow through our body. Therefore, Wisneski and Anderson use the chakra system and apply it to the biological model of science instead of going the other way around.

1.6 Mind and body experiment by Dr. Dispenza

According to Dr. Joe Dispenza it is easy to view the chakra system as an esoteric field of made-up beliefs without putting in effort to understand their theory regarding physiological impact on our body. On this basis he conducted his experiment where he explored the possibility of a connection between our mind and body. With a control group and an experimental group he used a meditation technique to see if there were any effects of the practice over a set span of time. During meditation he asked his subjects to envision enlarged biceps to note down if their biceps would increase in mass through a simple meditation routine.

By the end, Dr. Dispenza was able to measure a significant positive result in his experimental group. He noticed that his participants had grown an average of 25% mass around the bicep area[35]. In comparison to that, the control group did not show significant muscular growth. The conclusion of this research which produced similar results when repeated by other researchers, is that our thoughts can cause visible biochemical reactions in our body. In other words, we have the capability to control what type of chemical signals are sent to our body to produce a desired result. This research gives the chakra system a fact check since energy medicine is designed to strengthen the link between mind and body.

1.7 The endocrine system and chakras

The location of each energy center as described by the chakra theory corresponds majorly with specific glands found in our body that make up the endocrine system. This part of our anatomy is also dubbed as a 'biochemical powerhouse' because it regulates our bodily functions just like the chakras are supposed to. Certain researchers maintain that the chakra system is just another explanation of how our endocrine system functions and its purpose to maintain homeostasis as well as physiological balance in the body.

According to these authors, the root chakra is responsible for feeling grounded and secure. Just like that the adrenal gland is in charge of fight or flight response in times of a threating situation in order to maintain our innate need for physical survival. Similar to that, the sacral chakra is in charge of our emotional and sexual health. It is compared with our reproductive glands by researchers because these glands are supposed to be responsible of our sexual desires and reproduction. Other than this, the solar plexus chakra's definition is very close to pancreas found in mammals. This gland is present to make sure our organs in the abdomen such as kidneys, liver, and intestines are functioning in a healthy manner. Energy medicine scholars suggest that just like the pancreas should be healthy so that our organs are strong, the solar plexus chakra located near the stomach should be open and balanced to have the same physiological effects.

Furthermore, the heart chakra is associated with our thymus gland which regulates our immune system. The heart, lungs and blood system are majorly controlled by the thymus gland and any symptoms related to these organs can lead to heart disease and other problems. The side effects of our thymus gland are just like the drawbacks of unbalanced heart chakra. On a similar note, the throat chakra is thought to be a representation of our thyroid gland which regulates our metabolism and releases our hormones in our body for growth[36]. These researchers mainly mapped out the locations of the endocrine system and noticed that it overlaps the chakra chart. In addition to that, because their responsibilities are also similar it can be concluded that these ancient scholars were indeed describing a structure that is concrete in nature.

To sum up, while both psychology and medical science oppose the existence of the chakras system, these schools of thought can also be used to substantiate the claims made by energy medicine scholars. It can be said that the need to measure these energy channels is invalid because how empirical science and psychology describe human body and mind already overlaps with what the chakra system had theorized centuries ago. In that case, a mere application of already existing data can give this ancient theory the scientific support it needs.

CHAPTER 4

The Root Chakra

In the previous chapters we talked about how the chakra system is structured, its theory about human life and energy medicine. We also investigated whether the existence of this prehistoric meditation technique is supported by empirical science. After sufficient background information, we are now going to unfold what is included in the chakra system and each of the seven chakras will be explored in an orderly manner.

As we know, each chakra corresponds to a specific part of our bodies and defines the features we hold within us. As the first chakra of your body, the root chakra known as *Muladhara* in Sanskrit, plays a major role in your life and how you relate to the world around you. Our emotions are not just triggered by our mind but what resides physiologically in our bodies also has an effect on how we feel every day. Chakra scholars believe that this is because our body has the ability to communicate through these energy channels and certain energy messages are directly related to specific parts of our body. That is how we are able to tell which chakra needs to be strengthened and balanced.

LOCATION OF THE ROOT CHAKRA

As the first chakra of your body, this energy channel is located at the bottom of your body. Found near the end of your spine, chakra scholars point to the right side of the tailbone to identify the root chakra. Out of all seven chakras, this energy hub affects you physically the most. Yoga masters also suggest that this specific chakra is responsible for our primal need for survival and often dub it as 'the survival center'[37].

The reason why the root chakra is placed at the end of your spine is because chakra authors maintain that the vital life force energy that comes from this energy channel begins at the conception of babies. The cells divide during the embryogenesis stage and the spine begins to form from the bottom (the tailbone) and moves to the top where the crown chakra is located. After that, other organs begin to develop in the fetus.

The color of root chakra

As we all know, our chakras are not physically present and therefore they are invisible to the naked eye. This is the reason why these energy vortexes are assigned colors. However, each color of these chakras is also different because it holds certain characteristics of the specific chakra. In this case, the root chakra resonates with red because that is the color of our blood and it signifies our life force.

Adding to that analogy, the red color of this chakra also means that wearing red clothes, using red meditation, wearing red jewelry and so on floods your aura with red and aids you with aligning your root chakra with the entire system and revitalizes it. Red objects stimulate this chakra and if this color therapy is repeated in your everyday life your root chakra always stays balanced[38].

Significance of the Root Chakra

The color of this root chakra also gives it significance in the chakra system. On a biological level, the color red is linked with our adrenal gland which functions to resonate a fight or flight response when a situation linked to our survival occurs. As mentioned earlier, this is how the root chakra is associated with our instinct for survival. With that, because it is located near the lowest part of your body, it keeps us grounded and gives our life stability, meaning and a purpose. Chakra authors believe that it is our root chakra that connects our bodies with Earth and gives us a sense of the physical realm[39].

General Features of the Root Chakra

Often called the Earth chakra, the main features of this energy channel are stability in social and personal life, reliability, and development of thoughtfulness. Because this chakra is denoted by the element of Earth, this channel has a reputation for making people feel nurtured and whole. When your root chakra is functioning at its optimal level, you become self-accepting, supportive and peaceful towards yourself and others around you. The root chakra helps you find comfort in your skin and be okay with who you are.

The sense of being grounded helps us grow as a person and feel at home with ourselves and worry less about the negativity you often fixate on in your life. That is how the root chakra is responsible for our physical and emotional stability. Just like a plant, the stronger our root is, the bigger we are likely to bloom. That is the correlation that this chakra follows. Through these features, the root chakra gives us a solid foundation and helps us open the rest of our chakras. It is often emphasized by chakra scholars that without a balanced root chakra, working on the remaining chakras is nearly impossible. Based on this piece of information, imagine you are building a house where you will be living for a long time. Without a solid foundation built in firm soil with strong basic structure, the house is unlikely to be functional and instead it is more prone to falling down quickly. Just like that, the root chakra holds all the other chakras together and maintains the energy flow[40].

Other than this, the root chakra maintains your emotional health strictly by helping you let go of any underlying irrational fears. Because of these fears, you are more likely to stay stressed and worried every day which can interrupt your emotional and physical health. A healthy root chakra tackles this problem and makes you worry less as each day passes by. On the other hand, the root chakra is also responsible for your sense of worthiness. Similar to Erikson's stage of trust vs. mistrust that we analyzed in the previous chapter, those who were unable to find security in their childhood tend to become mistrustful of others around them. However, this sense of trust is brought back through a functional root chakra. This energy channel strengthens your sense of worth once it helps remove the effects of negative experiences in your life. These can include discouragement in childhood, abuse, lack of support as a child and so on.

A strong root chakra gives you balance in situations where you are at the risk of feeling anxious and overwhelmed. When you are confronted by a threatening place, person or event, your root chakra gives you the energy to focus and make the best decisions in these scenarios. With that, the root chakra is the cupid in your life. When this chakra manifests its energy, it helps you develop healthy and authentic human connections in the world. Instead of focusing on the people you want, the root chakra brings you closer to the people you need in your life to feel fulfilled[41]. In doing so, the root chakra strengthens your ability to have faith in yourself and others around you. Often people struggle with existential crisis because of their personal experiences. However, a healthy root chakra brings you closer to your highest human potential and that is how you find your purpose on this planet.

An Unbalanced Root Chakra

The best way to undergo root chakra therapy is by paying attention to how you feel, what you frequently think about and note down any irregular physical sensations you might be experiencing. However, for a beginner it is often confusing to notice the signs of an unhealthy root chakra. In that case, we have a list of signs that are often reported by disciples of chakra healing. What exactly is an unbalanced root chakra? The expected state of all your chakras is one where the energy is flowing without interruption. With that, the flow of this energy should not fluctuate and should remain at its optimal level. When a chakra becomes unbalanced it is likely that either something is blocking the energy flow entirely or the flow of energy has heightened instead of being distributed evenly among the remaining six chakras.

Signs of Unbalanced Root Chakra

- *Obsessing about money*; in case your root chakra is unbalanced your sense of financial security can be disrupted. You are more likely to begin worrying that you do not have enough money for survival and such catastrophic thoughts cloud your mind with stress about getting poor. You might also start overworking yourself to bring your anxiety down. This obsession can occur the other way around as well where you believe that only you can control the assets that you are supposed to share with your family.

- *An unbalanced root chakra can lead you to develop trust issues in your personal life;* you often become paranoid regarding the intentions of those around you. With that, such individuals also begin to distance themselves from people and feel lonely more often[42]. In addition to that, people suffering from an unbalanced root chakra believe that the only person that is reliable is them and a general mistrust of others is how they will be able to survive in the society.

- *Feeling nervous and anxious at all times*; Just like the previous analogy of a weak foundation, when your root chakra is blocked, it can lead you to feeling unstable in life often taking a toll on your self-confidence. You constantly think that you are incapable in terms of handling problems, impressing others around you, and you are least likely to succeed in both personal and professional life.

- *An unbalanced root chakra means heightened anger*; those who lose touch with their foundation often develop a habit of lashing out on others around them without a rational reason. They hold bitter grudges and feel they have been wronged without analyzing themselves in a particular situation[43].

- *'People walk all over me';* this thought is what frequently occurs in your head with your root chakra is blocked. You believe that people only notice you in order to get favors and this further makes you develop a fear regarding building relationships.

- *Bad eating habits;* A physical symptom of unhealthy root chakra is change in your eating routine. You might either begin to overeat or eat very less. This leads you to a dark path of developing serious health issues such as malnutrition, weak muscles, losing body mass or increasing body mass quickly, contracting viruses easily and becoming prone to other acute health issues. In addition to that, it drains your energy level and you always feel tired both mentally and physically.

- *Losing your sense of self;* because your root chakra is in charge of keeping you grounded, this feature gets interrupted once your chakra is unbalanced. Over time, people begin to lose their understanding of self and are unable to recognize who they are and what they want in life as well as their purpose of existence. This further makes them prone to serious mental disorders such as bad sleeping pattern, paranoia, split personality disorder and so on if the root chakra remains unhealed.

- *Physical signs of unbalanced root chakra*; when you suffer from a blocked root chakra you begin to suffer from various digestive problems due to the location of this chakra. You can notice symptoms like constipation, lower back pain, prostate problems, kidney stones and bladder issues[44].

ROOT CHAKRA HEALING MEDITATION

Did these symptoms of unhealthy root chakra alert you? Relax and take a deep breath because the good news is that there are several successful healing practices you can indulge in when you notice your first chakra is blocked. Over time, once you are able to develop an ability of firm concentration, you will begin to notice the changes in your symptoms. Feeling the reverse of these signs means that you are making progress and your root chakra has begun to shift back to its natural and healthy state.

1.1 Affirmation mantra

One of the best tools that you can use to heal the 'muladhara' is chanting a common affirmation mantra. For this technique, many individuals do not need external help and they can depend on their will power instead. This technique requires people to sit in a meditation space where they feel comfortable and repeat to themselves 'I am safe, I am secure'. An additional mantra to affirm your faith is 'the universe will provide me with whatever I need'. Repeating the mantra routinely will reopen your root chakra and get rid of the symptoms that are bringing you down.

1.2 Yoga Asana

Chakra authors suggest that practicing specific yoga positions can also help your root chakra. These specific poses from the asana chart include; Padmasana (lotus flexion), Pavanamuktasana (knee to chest position), Malasana (squatting pose), and Sirsanana (head to knee pose). For beginners who do not practice yoga, it is advised to work under a yoga practitioner first in order to make sure the healing practice is working in favor of your root chakra.

1.3 Aromatherapy

The good thing about this chakra system is that the ways to open your root chakra do not cost you a fortune. Chakra healers believe that the essence of sandalwood, rosewood, ginger, cloves, cedar, black pepper, and rosemary can help you heal your root chakra. For this therapy, you are not required to put in much energy except maintain relaxed state of mind during aromatherapy. During this type of meditation, you can also apply oils on your body to heal this chakra[45].

1.4 Crystal therapy

Germs are very popular for healing the root charka. Because this energy channel is assigned the red color, the stones that correspond to its energy are red jasper, bloodstone, citrine, carnelian, Smokey quartz, black tourmaline, azurite, and obsidian. Simply placing any of these stones on your body during a meditation session helps you absorb their energy and tune your root chakra with your body.

1.5 Sound therapy

Chakra authors believe that the root chakra vibrates like the 'C' note found in music language. Due to this characteristic, certain types of music can help you open your root chakra. During a chakra meditation, you can put on chants and music dominated with the 'C' note and focus on feeling the vibrations flow through your body. This awakens a relax state of mind which is beneficial for rewiring your root chakra. Root chakra meditational music tracks are easily available in this digital world and you can often find them free of charge[46].

ROOT CHAKRA GUIDED MEDITATION
BRINGING BALANCE TO THE ROOT CHAKRA

Before you start with a guided meditation, there are a few personal changes that will contribute to a healthy recovery of your lower chakra:

1. Practice grounding exercises; this daily routine technique requires you to concentrate and feel the 'rooting' of your feet to the ground.
2. Change in diet; eating food items such as carrots, beets, apples, and turnips can give you an extra boost.
3. Embrace the nature; in order to get rid of your daily stress you can opt for walking barefoot in your lawn or a nearby park.

Meditation Guide

- Sit in a chair with your feet flat on the ground. Any position in which you can maintain comfortably during the meditation is suitable.

- Even when you meditate it is okay to have thoughts but don't strain yourself while trying to get rid of them. Simply be gentle to yourself and bring yourself back to attention in case your thoughts take you somewhere else.

- Lastly, if you have any expectations you should brush them off. Instead of staying calculated, invest your time in the calm and silence.

Beginning the session:

Once you are sitting in a comfortable position, close your eyes.

Balance Your Chakras

Slowly bring awareness towards your normal breathing.

As the concentration builds you will begin to notice the rise and fall of your upper body.

In case you have thoughts wandering in, take your time and come back to the meditation gently.

Now you will take three deep breaths.

Bring your attention to the deep breathing and notice the natural rhythm it creates.

Now it is time to move deeper into the chakra meditation. Bring your attention to the base of your spine. This is the location of your root chakra.

Try to imagine this energy center as a crimson light pin in your mind.

As you keep taking deep breaths, imagine the size of this red light pin growing slowly.

With another breath, let the red light envelop your lower body. Imagine it surrounding your body.

In your imagination let this ruby light be around you for a few moments and then send it towards your feet.

Balance Your Chakras

Focus on your breath and concentrate on your imagination and you will feel grounded as you get in touch with the sensation of the flour beneath you.

Once your feet are relaxed, imagine the light moving to your legs. Let it relax your muscles.

After that, imagine the red light move up towards your hip bones and thighs. Take a couple of deep breaths and let it calm you.

Now the light will expand to your lower spine. As you imagine this crimson light surrounding your lower body, you will take a deep breath and concentrate on your blood pumping.

There is no strict time limit for this meditation. You can end your session once it helps you feel relaxed and grounded.

CHAPTER 5

The Sacral Chakra

Now that we know everything we need to understand about the root chakra, it's time to move forward to the second energy house in your body. The sacral chakra helps you add a little spice in your life. It offers you access to the three 'Fs'; fun, flexibility, and flow. In working with this energy vortex, you will be able to address the type of relationship you have with others around you and yourself as well. Once the chakra opens, you will be able to discover the ultimate powers you have within your body.

With that, sacral chakra meditation will aid you in cultivating a healthy relationship with seeking pleasure. We all know how hard it can be to let yourself be rewarded without any underlying guilt. In addition to that, once you refine your knowledge about the sacral chakra you will gain insight into your deepest emotions and secrets. At the end of your sacral chakra healing journey, you will master the art of expressing yourself skillfully and you will find the courage to set strong boundaries.

FACTS ABOUT THE SACRAL CHAKRA

The sacral chakra is located behind the pelvis. This chakra is above the root chakra and below your solar plexus chakra. The name comes from its correspondence to the sacrum found in your spine. Resonating with the music note D, this energy house is assigned the color orange because orange is a color for warmth, protection, and creativity.

Yoga scholars believe that our emotions reside physically in our bodies. In that case, the second chakra focuses on letting an individual discover their hobbies, create things they love, build exciting relationships and embrace their sexual eroticism. Centered towards our personal identity, this energy channel helps you take off the mask you wear in public and be your real self. With that, an individual is able to form harmonious friendships and long-lasting relationships in life.

Due to its location, the second chakra is deeply rooted within our sexual lives[47]. Chakra scholars often dub it as 'the pleasure chakra' because it helps us stay connected to our partnerships in life. However, sexual expression is just one form of the emotional and physical freedom this chakra provides us with. As pleasure can be associated with numerous things in life, it simply helps you engage in the physical things you enjoy in life such as fishing, writing poetry, painting and so on. Additionally, by giving us liberation from our fear of accepting happiness through human experience it lets you get in touch with your spirituality.

The sacral chakra teaches us about the power each one of us holds within us. With a healthy second chakra, you are able to realize what you want in your life. Once that is taken care of, you begin to utilize your talent and express the life you want to live.

Another important lesson individuals get from the role of sacral chakra is how to create relationships in life; starting from casual engagements to the most intimate partnerships. A healthy sacral chakra removes anything toxic you have learnt about relationships and resets the definitions attached with it. You learn how to process pain through your sacral chakra. With that, you become aware of your wrongdoings and any karma that might be linked to it. If a relationship does not work out, instead of attacking yourself you are able to learn from its limitations and grow as a person. On the other hand, the sacral chakra is also connected to your sexual health and well-being. A balanced second chakra aids women with sexual gratification as well as the process of giving birth without complications. Because of its location, the organs around the pelvis in both men and women are its responsibility[48].

UNBALANCED SACRAL CHAKRA SIGNS

In case you are struggling with an unhealthy lifestyle, all fingers are pointed towards your sacral chakra. The key to restoring balance in your second chakra is familiarizing yourself with the indications of a blocked or overactive sacral chakra. Most of the symptoms of an overactive sacral chakra express themselves in a non-physical manner however, there are a handful of physical symptoms you might encounter as well.

Due to unbalanced activity in your sacral chakra you might feel n constant warm sensation in your lower body. This happens because the flow of energy in this channel is excessive. This also impacts the functions of your lower back, reproductive organs and the bladder. The most common physical expressions of the sacral chakra include lower back pain, cysts in ovaries, urinary issues, unhealthy kidneys, and other gynecological problems.

Because your sacral chakra is in an overwhelming state, it might lead you towards weakening your personal boundaries and become excessively dependent on others with a potential of becoming obsessive in nature. The emotional downsides of an unbalanced sacral chakra also include heightened aggression, anxiety, arrogance, and mania. When there is over activity in this chakra, it can cause emotional over-reactions meaning becoming clingy towards people and/or forming emotional attachments with objects. With a lot of co-dependency on relationships, overactive sacral energy also makes you feel detached, promiscuous, and a sex addict. You might begin to view others as mere vessels for your sexual gratification instead of forming a wholesome relationship[49].

People with an unbalanced sacral chakra are also at risk of developing substance abuse, alcohol dependency, and constantly engaging in risky life experiences. With that, a blockage in this chakra can either lead you to eating disorders such as binging and/or body dysmorphic disorder. Also known as the navel chakra, it governs your ability to be flexible and adapt the community around you. However, if this chakra is out of control it can take a toll on your ability to interact with others, nurture relationships, and define your life.

An unbalanced sacral chakra takes away your ability to stay focused. With a lack of attention, an individual's mind is inclined to be consumed by fantasies that distract them from confronting their problems and working on them. Slowly, people begin to misplace their sense of community and lose themselves in their dream world. As a blocked sacral chakra takes a toll on your ability to turn your ideas into action, it also decreases your ability to be creative. If you notice yourself lacking passion for hobbies you used to enjoy, it is best to take it as a hint and start sacral chakra healing.

SACRAL CHAKRA MEDITATION TECHNIQUES

There are specific techniques that can heal your sacral chakra and take the uneasiness away from your body. As meditation can be time-consuming, on days when you have to be on the go, you can opt for **crystal healing**. There are numerous orange gemstones that you can carry on yourself in a form of sacral chakra jewelry. While you can go with any precious stone of yoru choice, there are four gemstones that scholars highly recommend.

- **Orange Calcite:** This sacral chakra healing stone enhances your creativity, break emotional barriers and sharpens your mind-body connection

- **Moonstone:** As it comes in various colors, this stone in peach color stimulates your mind. IT reduces your worries and adds a loving energy in your atmosphere

- **Carnelian:** This semi-precious stone in reddish-brown works magic by helping you discover your artsy and creative side.

- **Citrine:** This golden yellow stone is guaranteed for increasing your self-esteem especially when you experience reduced confidence due to sacral chakra imbalance.

In addition to crystal healing, there are various **sacral chakra affirmations** that you can repeat to yourself when you are meditating. As you continue with your routine you will be able to reduce the time it takes you to concentrate and align your chakra. Sit in a relaxed position and close your eyes. Once you are able to build concentration you can begin your meditation by repeating any of the following affirmations[50]. You can even make combinations of these chants and notice if the customization works for your routinely healing:

- I am deserving of a pleasure-filled experience and my needs should be met.

- I am confident in what I offer the world and it is enough.

- Expressing my sexual self in healthy, fun and creative ways is a safe practice.

- I'm capable of attracting loving, good, and supportive people.

- I'm capable of embracing change and making the best out of my future.

- Every day is for experiencing joy and satisfaction.

- I have the potential for creation and I am full of inspiration.

- My body is vibrant and I find comfort in it.
- I'm capable of giving love and receiving love.

Sacral Chakra Guided Meditation

It is important to remember that sacral chakra healing cannot be done by only depending on meditation routines. Instead you have to take care of your physical body to produce emotional reactions that boost your chakra. The following items come highly recommended by scholars:

- **Oranges:** This fruit helps align your sacral chakra with the rest of your energy channels. Other fleshy food items that can give you an extra push include mangoes, peaches, and papayas.

- **Seeds:** Chakra scholars always advise their disciples to eat seeds such as sunflower, poppy, hemp, and pumpkin to heal your sacral chakra.

- **Cocoanuts:** Coconuts consist of various healthy oils and fats that give you energy. They're a popular choice among people wanting to create the right mood to showcase their creative side.

- **Teas:** Clear liquids are said to be beneficial for healing your second chakra which is why fruit tea is an excellent choice for opening the sacral chakra[51].

Meditation guide:

Before we begin with our meditation script for sacral chakra, there are three things you must remember:

- When our chakras are out of balance we often begin to question our place on this Earth. Grounding exercises are built to help you rekindle that connection with this planet.

- The stress that you get from removing your thoughts is not healthy for your healing. In that case, let them be in your mind and slowly let them fade away.

- In the rush of achieving what everyone else is, do not forget to spend some time by yourself and the nature around you.

Meditation script

Are you tired after having a long day? You might have begun to lose your confidence in the things you create. It's important to remember that it's impossible to always remain composed. Everyone is capable of getting a little out of the line and a little self-help can put you right back on the track. Now, let's begin with sacral chakra meditation to remove any negative thoughts you have brought back home with you. As they pile up, they can put your sacral chakra out of balance.

Sit in a comfortable and quiet place. Don't get overwhelmed and take ten slow breaths.

Once you are able to feel a little relaxed, close your eyes. Take another deep breath.

Visualization needs concentration but it is okay to let your thoughts wonder. Let them slowly fade away with the deep breaths you take. Once you have a clear head, it's time to get creative.

Picture a spinning orange circle around your sacral chakra. These rays of orange are spreading out in rippling waves and slowly surrounding your whole body. You can start to feel the warmth it brings to you.

Once the visualization is strong, keep taking deep breaths. Continue the practice for as long as it takes for you to feel calm.

Channeling the energy of your chakra in your imagination awakens it eventually and brings balance to your sacral chakra. Finish the practice by slowly opening your eyes. Take five deep breaths after.

CHAPTER 6

Solar Plexus Chakra

In life we experience the good and the bad. Good energy helps us become a better person but the negative energy can take a toll on us. As having strength is necessary for survival sometimes the bad things wear us out and it is hard to get a clear picture of life. However, many of us only realize when the situation blocks the flow of our life. In that case, how do you know if there is any emotional blockage that is stopping you from moving forward in life? Most of us carry the weight and these blockages can show up anywhere; at work and/or relationships.

We always have a gut feeling that something is not adding up. Sooner or later we discover the truth about ourselves when the negative experiences begin to create an imbalance in our mind, body and spirit. The first step is to recognize where an energy block has occurred and learn which chakras need their energy restored. Here we will begin with our third chakra; the solar plexus chakra. This cleverly structured information will aid you on your journey to self-healing.

FUNCTIONS OF THE SOLAR PLEXUS CHAKRA

The solar plexus chakra can be found above the navel and below the sternum. The functions of this energy channel are associated with our ego. In order words, the solar plexus chakra is a channel for self-belief, personal power, and self-worth. When this chakra is activated you always find courage to do something that is scary for you. Moreover, you find the confidence in you to speak for yourself. Individuals with a healthy solar plexus chakra are not afraid to exert self-control and willpower.

When you are in such situations with a balanced solar plexus chakra you will notice that you have control over yourself, you are commanding, you have a firm voice and your posture is powerful. This personal power that solar plexus chakra boosts does not mean exerting power over others instead it refers to self-mastery. You achieve the ability to master processing of your thoughts and emotions. By controlling these two aspects you overcome fear and make appropriate decisions in any situation.

The solar plexus chakra is assigned the color yellow because it empowers you to follow your path without any distractions[52]. With that, the vibrant yellow color is associated with the qualities of intellect, personality, ego, and creativity. Noted by the element of fire, this chakra brings clarity to your mind. Often a situation calls for a judgement. Such a responsibility can put a strain on us and make us anxious. When that happens there are higher chances for making a decision based on a clouded mindset. Though, when your solar plexus chakra is in full bloom it sharpens your decision-making skills.

The solar plexus chakra is also responsible for our expression of will. It provides you with a momentum to march forward in life and meet your goals without lagging behind because of temporary distractions. On this journey, it also helps you realize what your personal desires are and restrains you from neglecting them. Keeping you on the right direction in life, it makes sure that you don't forget your morals. This energy channel fuels your spirit to work on your social status and how to behave in a community. With the power of solar plexus chakra individuals are able to tell the difference between what is defined as right and wrong according to their society's standards.

Additionally, this chakra controls your interpretation of criticism from other people[53]. When the societal feedback makes you think you are not good enough, this energy vortex stops you from bringing yourself down. You learn lessons from difficult situations and maintain your independence regardless.

SYMPTOMS OF UNBALANCED SOLAR PLEXUS CHAKRA

Now that you understand what lies on the shoulders of your solar plexus chakra we should take a glance at what happens to your body and emotions when this chakra is blocked. The commonly reported solar plexus problems can grow as the nature of this chakra deteriorates further. Although, these symptoms are easy to notice because most of them hinder how you perform in your daily life and around your community.

When your solar plexus chakra is out of balance you feel the need to control everything and every person around you. While it is a quality this energy channel helps you unlock, it can also backfire. Blocked or overflowing energy chakra takes away your ability to co-operate and work together. Instead you become overly concerned with making things go your way. In that case, you develop a need to exert dysfunctional control over people. This drive for control also comes from feeling helpless. A weak solar plexus chakra disrupts your thought process and makes you think that no one has your back. You lose faith in people and begin to believe that you can only trust yourself to get results.

Furthermore, blockage of the solar plexus channel makes it difficult for individuals to see the big picture in life[54]. As we grow up what we want in our future becomes clear to us. This shapes our life's purpose and direction we take to meet the goal(s) we have set. Nonetheless, when this energy house is out of balance it brings an existential crisis with it. In this state of mind it becomes extremely difficult for us to hope for a future that satisfies us. When this symptom comes into play, it lowers your self-esteem as a side-effect.

Dreams that once brought excitement to you become blurry and you become consumed by any unsettled guilt from your past. If the blockage is minor it can reduce your ambitiousness and confidence in one part of your life. Meanwhile, if the level of imbalance increases the negative effects become universal.

While the emotional symptoms are a lot to handle, people eventually develop physical side effects. Due to the location of this chakra, these symptoms are concerned with your digestive system. General public reports having acute digestive cramps without any medical cause. When these symptoms are left untreated for a while they result in bloating of your stomach and nausea. A person's eating habits also get out of control; either individuals over-indulge in food, eat unhealthy or they consume less calories than they need. Over-time, the imbalance causes your short-term memory to weaken as well. Although if you read the signs timely you can prevent a significant block.

MEDITATION TECHNIQUES

There are several ways that you can use to open your solar plexus chakra. Often individuals go for a simple meditation that relaxes their body and mind. However, adding a combination is necessary to awaken your solar plexus chakra. You can either pick one of the following or more to turn your daily meditation routine into solar plexus chakra healing process:

1. **Wear yellow and eat yellow:** Because yellow vibrates solar plexus chakra's energy change in your diet and wardrobe choices can slowly bring the balance back.

2. **Exercise:** Any amount and sort of physical exertion on your body is suitable for the optimization of the third chakra.

3. **Gemstone meditation:** Yellow crystals such as tiger's eye, yellow topaz, and yellow tourmaline align your solar plexus chakra. Simply place this gemstone near your navel and meditate for healing to take place.

4. **Tattoos:** The sign for solar plexus chakra includes a flower with ten petals and a triangle in the middle occasionally. Those who are open to body art are encouraged to get this tattoo to resonate their third chakra.

5. **Practice yoga:** Before you begin meditation you can indulge in some morning yoga and/or dance routine to heal this chakra[55].

SOLAR PLEXUS CHAKRA MEDITATION SCRIPT

In order to fuel your solar plexus chakra with energy and remove any blockages there are several lifestyle changes that chakra scholars offer their disciples:

Celebrate victories: While you are on your journey never take yourself for granted. Whether your achievement(s) was minor or major you should celebrate it routinely.

Mirror exercises: If you feel confident in yourself sit in front of a mirror and see yourself. During this meditation as you manage to hold on to a calm interior you will be able to connect with yourself spiritually. Look past your physical body and search for your soul.

Treat yourself: No one knows us better than ourselves and what we need. From time to time, you should reward yourself. Maybe you should purchase those shoes you had your eye on since fall. These spiritual practices give you an emotional boost and help you feel special.

While we have given you additional tips and tricks to unclog your sacral chakra, beginners can always make use of as much help as they can get. In that case, the following is a short script you can stick to when you engage in solar plexus chakra meditation:

> For many beginners meditation can be more exhausting than calming. Although, adding a bit of fun only brings out positive results. In that case, let's begin by sitting in a comfortable position in a space that makes you feel safe.

After settling down, observe the space around you. Capture the atmosphere, the temperature, the lights and sound around you.

Take as much time as you need to unwind.

Now that you have familiarized yourself to the space, close your eyes.

Take five deep breaths and calm your nerves.

Let the wandering thoughts take their time to go away and do not exert pressure on yourself.

Are you relaxed yet? In that case, let's begin with our version of a funky dance solar plexus chakra meditation.

Start by concentrating on how your body feels. Take deep breaths as you go forward.

Once you have connected with your body, slowly begin to stand. If you notice your concentration breaking, you can take soothing breaths to bring yourself back.

Now that you have gotten up, close your eyes again and maintain the composure.

Getting in touch with your bodily sensations must make you feel grounded. This is the best time to begin our dance and visualization meditation.

As you feel free in your body, you can begin to sway your body. Stay calm and move in directions that you naturally feel like.

Swing your arms around freely and slowly take your focus away from how your body is moving.

As you find peace in making humble movements, it is time to start with the visualization. In case you need to pause for some time, you can proceed to do so.

As your body sways, visualize an image. It's a figurative representation of your solar plexus chakra. It's a yellow light surrounding your body. Imaging this vibrates with your chakra and slowly opens it.

The yellow light is surrounding your whole body as you let it sway. It is wrapped around you.

Slowly shift this yellow ray towards your feet. Let it stay there for a minute.

Now this yellow light is moving towards your legs. Sway and hold the visualization for another minute.

In the next minute, this yellow light will move towards your lower abdomen where the solar plexus chakra is placed. Now you will hold this position for the remainder of time.

As your imagination becomes stronger, it's time to slowly end your meditation.

Remain calm and indulge in the meditation session for as long as it takes to ease your mind and body.

Once you have unlocked tranquility, slowly stop the dance and open your eyes.

Sit down in a comfortable position and take five deep breaths. End the session eventually.

CHAPTER 7

The Heart Chakra

There has been a great debate about whether or not our emotions are connected to how our body feels. When it comes down to it, chakra scholars have always believed that inside the human body emotions reside physically. When you focus more on this analogy, it can be concluded that our emotions are an expression of what goes on inside our bodies. In order to listen to our body attention needs to be paid to the emotions we are experiencing. Certain energetic jolts are directly linked to specific parts of our body and it can affect the state of our chakras.

The chakra system is our weapon for handling challenges in our life. Through the phases of our chakras we gather an in-depth understanding of our personal power. Considering that, if your heart chakra is out of balance think of it as an experience that will make you stronger. With this chapter, you will be able to unlock the signs of a healthy heart chakra and symptoms of an imbalanced heart chakra. Once this knowledge becomes your tool you will be able to focus better on the recommended therapies for heart chakra.

FUNCTIONS OF HEART CHAKRA

Before understanding the various functions of a healthy heart chakra, you should always make note of some of its key attributes. The first characteristic of the heart chakra is its location. This energy house is placed in the middle of your chest. Beginners often confuse the whereabouts of this chakra and believe that it lies where our heart is. However, as mentioned earlier the reality is slightly different than that. Secondly, the heart chakra is noted by the color green. If the energy in this chakra is high then the color can turn to pink. Although, normally the aura of heart chakra is denoted by shades of green.

In addition to that, just like all seven chakras, this one has its special symbol too. According to chakra scholars, the symbol for this energy hub includes two intersecting triangles that form a six-sided star surrounded by a circle with twelve petals. Lastly, the heart chakra is directly linked to the element of air[56]. This defines the waves of energy this chakra holds. Associated with our breath, this chakra's energy represents the ideas of spaciousness and connection with all things around us.

The heart chakra is a central powerhouse of our body. It acts as a bridge that connects the root chakra, sacral chakra, and solar plexus chakra with the remaining three chakras found in the upper body of a human being. With such a responsibility, the heart chakra can be understood as a mediator between our spirit and body. This energy channel fuels the health and strength of these two elements. While this is an important function of the heart chakra, there are various other properties related to this energy house.

The heart chakra directly influences our emotion of love. Known as *Anahata* in Sanskrit, this chakra deals with our ability to accept and give unconditional love to ourselves and those around us. Love is the greatest emotional power a human has. However, due to our personal experiences often we never learn what unconditional love means and how it makes an individual feel. Nevertheless, your heart chakra provides you with something you might lack because of your external environment. With its ability to teach us what unconditional love is, the heart chakra propels us to work on our emotional development. It gives us the wisdom to learn healthy ways of expressing love and compassion.

Additionally, the heart chakra brings us closer to innocence. As children we are able to react to a situation with different emotions such as love, hope, fear, confidence and so on. However, as adults the transparency of emotional expression starts clouding due to exposure to extremely challenging situations. But with the help of the heart chakra, this child-like innocence comes back to us. We become capable of acceptance and forgiveness.

Instead of holding onto grudges and biases, we gain the quality of letting go of the negativity and keeping an open mind[57]. The heart chakra also teaches us how to process grief without denial and/or repression. The energy it radiates helps us find peace within us and share it with other individuals. As the heart chakra is located in your chest it is also responsible for your cardiac system and respiratory system. These interdependent organs rely on air to function properly. In such a way the gland thymus is also under the primary care of the heart chakra. When the fourth chakra stays balanced our immune system is regulated and hormone production continues to give us physical strength without any flaws.

How to spot an unbalanced heart chakra

Just like the previous three chakras, your heart chakra is capable of either being blocked, unblocked, or closed. These three states only occur when emotional and physical strains pile up and disrupt the natural flow of energy through this door. This universal energy flows through our vessels to maintain our emotions, physical health and soul on a spiritual plane. In case your heart chakra has gotten old and rusty, there are a few clear signs that you can watch out for. When you catch the culprit you will be able to apply the right therapeutic technique(s) and balance your fourth chakra to absorb its beneficial energy again.

Things such as emotional pain and stress often come from bad memories, a damaged child-parent relationship, overthinking, and repressing experiences that need to be confronted and dealt with[58]. Over time the negativity makes it difficult for you to establish and maintain healthy relationships. If left untreated for a while, eventually your heart chakra can become blocked or overcharged. In that case, do not forget to stay connected to yourself and pay attention to your emotions, habits, and thoughts. The first sign of an imbalance in heart chakra is disruption in your love life. We all have had a significant relationship from our past that we had to get over in order to move forward. However, when your heart chakra is blocked you seem to dwell over someone from the past and over time you get stuck in that state of mind. Individuals lack the motivation to get out of this rut and focus on building other healthy relationships.

With a fixation on a previous relationship, you also begin to hold grudges against your friends and family instead of letting things go and putting your mind at ease. Grudges are universal and it is okay to hold on to them only if you intend to let it go. Although, those struggling with a blocked heart chakra hold on to the pain and keep away from experiencing joy. As you go down this rabbit hole, the imbalance affects your ability to trust people. Whether it is a romantic relationship or a platonic friendship you become overwhelmed with the fear of betrayal. As a result, people begin to doubt others and it often leads to hurtful conversations.

As the toxicity due to blocked heart chakra grows, it begins to attack you on a personal level. Are you experiencing lack of confidence and low self-esteem? While no one is immune from these feelings from time to time, if they become frequent you should take it as a sign. Individuals start with becoming shy and keeping to themselves. Later, they become overly critical of their capabilities and qualities. Such a magnified lens on self leads to another negative effect of a blocked heart chakra. Attacking yourself frequently can lead you to bottle up your emotions. Finding a safe space to release your emotions is always best to sort this out. However, the blues that come with a blocked fourth chakra lead us to believe that no one wants to listen to us. Furthermore, overthinking and experiencing mood swings can become so intense that the only option an individual sees is repression of what is harming them. While you deal with the emotional side effects of a blocked heart chakra, your body weakens as well. Due to less energy, your immune system weakens and you become prone to catching infections and diseases. Prolonged blocked heart chakra can cause cardiac problems and breathing issues. With that, individuals suffer from hormonal imbalance too.

THERAPEUTIC REMEDIES FOR HEART CHAKRA

For thousands of years, the heart chakra has remained famous for helping us find our better half and balance in life. Although, when was the last time you were able to feel forgiveness, acceptance, generosity, connections, and love for yourself and others around you? This was probably the time when your heart chakra was still in balance. While this self-analysis question might have made you self-conscious, there is nothing to get anxious about. When something goes wrong with your body, there are always numerous ways to reverse that effect. If you think you have had enough and you would like to get rid of your chronic experiences of self-isolation, loneliness, resentment and bitterness, now is your time to take matters in your own hands. Following are several therapies that go in favor of rebalancing your heart chakra:

- **Love-kindness meditation:** The most beautiful feeling is a balanced heart chakra. It dissolves the illusions we create for ourselves and connects us with love. If you have the symptoms of a congested heart chakra, these remedies might just help you out. To do this meditation, sit down in a quiet room and concentrate on your breath. As you relax, think of things that you love about yourself to channel this energy towards yourself. Once that is done, think of four different people and note the things you love about them to direct this energy towards them. End the session when you are fulfilled.

- **Use herbs:** Other than meditation dietary additions can also open your heart chakra. Herbs such as nettle, hops, angelic, holy basil, rose and hawthorn clear the fourth chakra from any blockages. You can either add them to your food or drink them as herbal tea.

- **Yoga with crystals:** As we already know, these gemstones hold the energy that can rewire our chakras. Since there are specific crystals for each chakra, scholars have a whole list of gemstone recommendations to open your heart chakra. The best ones include green stones such as jade, emerald, rose quartz, rhodonite, green fluorite, ruby and prehnite. Simply place a combination of gemstones around you to absorb their energy while you do your daily yoga.

- While you indulge in these techniques you also need to make emotional and behavioral changes to continue with opening your heart chakra successfully. Chakra scholars suggest you can start by some of the following adjustments[59]:

- **Show yourself gratitude:** It's unfortunate how we take so much for granted in our life including ourselves. But one simple change that can rebalance your heart chakra is acknowledging the blessings you have in life. Sit down with a warm cup of herbal tea and think of all the things that helped you grow in life from time to time.

- **As 'What If':** Another self-adjustment that you need to make is practicing empathy. It is easier to make rash judgments about yourself and others than to remain optimistic and kind. The next time you find yourself in this situation, as yourself 'what if?'; For example, you are angry at another person and in that situation instead of attacking that person negatively you can ask yourself questions like 'what if that person was having a bad day?'.

- **Physical affection:** We are social creatures who require physical contact to feel safe, healthy and loved. Instead of withholding affection due to irrational thoughts try to engage in more hugs when you see your loved ones. Eventually, expressing love can help you attract love and kindness. While you are on it, give yourself a hug too when you're down!

Meditation Guide

What can you do to heal yourself when you also have to go outside and make a living? People with a busy schedule do not lack the motivation to take care of themselves but because there is so much on their plate, they are rarely able to focus on getting better. However, while in the previous years there might not have been a solution for this, we have the best suggestion now all thanks to technology. In case you are a 'Type A' personality and you cannot leave your busy schedule behind, you can rebalance your heart chakra as you start your routine every morning.

To begin with this meditation, there is a pre-plan that you need to work on. You will be making a heart chakra healing self-affirmation tape for your morning runs. Take some time out from your weekend and sit down to do some fun recordings. If you have an advanced mobile phone, you can make this recording directly. If the case is otherwise, a tape recorder will do the job.

After figuring out which mode you will use to record this tape, sit in a quiet place and make sure there is no other noise but yours. Take a few deep breaths and practice these affirmations offline to pronounce each word smoothly. When you are done, start the recording. In this tape, you will be adding some affirmations for the heart chakra. The following is a list you can choose from[60]:

- I am worthy of pure love.
- I direct love and kindness towards myself.
- My heart radiates powerful green rays.
- I love myself unconditionally.
- I am grateful for my blessings.
- I am open to receiving love and giving love.
- I choose to see myself in a positive light.
- My heart is free from hurt.

Now that you have all the material you need, you can start your heart chakra meditation while you get your daily exercise.

After you get ready for your morning walk or run, make sure to grab your affirmation tape along.

The reason why you recorded this is so that you can hear yourself say the things you must admit to. This powerful technique will resonate your clogged heart chakra over time.

Now that you are ready to start your morning workout, take five deep breaths first.

Feel yourself calming down. It's a nice and quiet morning and you are in your favorite jogging spot. Think of it as a regular day.

Once you have relaxed, hit the play button. Adjust the volume according to how you like it.

Don't rush with your jog/walk. Take your time. As you look around, slowly start to focus on the affirmations in the tape.

Take five calming breaths and repeat each affirmation to yourself. Repeat this cycle for at least twenty to thirty minutes of your jog/walk till you feel relaxed.

Chanting these affirmations will rebalance the greenlight of your heart chakra slowly because they will bring control back in your life.

CHAPTER 8

The Throat Chakra

Each chakra in our body has its own unique purpose. These energy houses make our living standard prime. Each day we have to face a new challenge in our familial life as well as our work. As every human possesses good qualities and bad qualities, these healthy chakras maintain a balance to help us function properly in our daily lives. Although, if any setbacks are not processed in a timely manner, they can pile up and hold us back.

Humans are meant to grow and learn as years pass by them. The direction of life and time is forward. But when the weight of our emotional baggage increases, this disrupts the chakras. As a result, our life becomes dysfunctional and hits a growth plateau. Now it's time to move forward to the fifth chakra in our body; the throat chakra. With our help, beginners will attain a clear picture of what a healthy throat chakra must feel like. Additionally, you can learn how to clear the channel if there seems to be a halt in the energy flow.

SIGNIFICANCE OF THROAT CHAKRA

As we move upward on the human anatomical figure chart, we can locate the chakra at the back of the neck. To be more specific, this energy channel is near the throat and it passes energy up and down from the lowest part of our body to the head. The function behind this energy flow is to help us express and communicate. According to chakra scholars, this energy house has many names. In Sanskrit the throat chakra is often called 'Vishudda', 'Kanth Padma', and 'Shodash Dala'. These words most commonly translate to 'pure' and 'purification'.

Because of the location of throat chakra it is associated with the pharyngeal as well as brachial plexus. In addition to that, the throat chakra is also connected to our jaws, tongue, palate, and mouth[61]. As it resonates with pure energy, the throat chakra also takes care of our neck and shoulders. If the throat chakra is healthy, it regulates our body temperature, growth, and metabolism. The thyroid gland is found near the throat and this chakra makes sure the growth hormones are being produced smoothly.

The symbol for throat chakra is made up of a circle with exactly sixteen petals on the side. Inside this circle is a crescent and sometimes the throat chakra symbol includes a triangle inscribed in another circle. Often the color of these petals is depicted by chakra scholars as grayish-lavender. This opens a discussion about the color of throat chakra. Scholars represent the throat chakra with blue, turquoise and sometimes as dark purple when the energy is high.

While these are the physical characteristics of the throat chakra, there are various emotional functions ascribed to this channel of energy. A healthy throat chakra is a house of expression. It gives us our ability to speak for ourselves and share our truth with others around us. When we are able to express our thoughts and concerns without hiding anything it strengthens our skill of communication. While verbal communication is throat chakra's specialty it also regulates our non-verbal communication skills. A functional throat chakra helps us be honest with ourselves and other individuals about what we are feeling, thinking, and desiring in life.

Another trait of the throat chakra is building a connection between our mind and spirit. As it is located near the throat, this chakra is often called the 'bottleneck' of energy movement in our body by scholars. When this channel is open, it aligns our spiritual visions with the reality we build. As that happens, we are able to use our intuition in our daily lives for protection and safety. In addition to that, yogis also mention that the throat chakra has a perfect template for other dimensions of the human body.

The throat chakra gives us the power to create what our life is going to be about[62]. With the help of its energy, humans are able to project their ideas into the real world. Our goals shift from fiction to reality and we get the satisfaction of feeling fulfilled in life. With that, the throat chakra also helps us realize which field we would like to get into when it comes to vocational life. For example, if you are an artist from within the throat chakra will help you acknowledge your talents and make the best of it. As the throat chakra is also concerned with the quality of our work life, it gives us our sense of timing. Individuals with a highly functional throat chakra are very good at time management and meeting deadlines. They refrain from lagging behind and always get their work done.

UNBALANCED THROAT CHAKRA SYMPTOMS

The wheel of life is supposed to distribute energy throughout our body so that any negative effects are kept away. Think of the chakra system as antibodies that remain activated in order to keep the bad bugs far away. However, stress, emotional drowning, mental conflict and anxiety are always a result of blockages in our chakra system. As these channels are interconnected when one falls down, the others get affected as well. The result of this dysfunction is mental, physical and spiritual suffering.

Just like that, when the throat chakra is imbalanced it can take a toll on our emotional and physical health. As individuals we are always working on our personal development. In order to do that we stay true to ourselves and keep away from distorted reality. We work on our communication to make sure our life is balanced and we also listen to others to make sure we regulate our behavior when it is needed. This is how humans are able to keep their world together.

When the throat chakra is underactive it means that the energy flow is not in equilibrium. As a result, our body can suffer physically. Both men and women can develop fever when the temperature is not regulated and if left untreated they can become immunocompromised. A healthy throat chakra is meant to protect the thyroid gland and aid in human body growth. However, when this chakra becomes congested it does not regulate the production of growth hormone. Many individuals also become prone to developing thyroid disease that can eventually be life-threatening. If the throat chakra suffers without any attempt at treatment it can go under trauma. A physical expression of throat chakra trauma is slurred speech.

There are also various behavioral and emotional side effects of an imbalanced throat chakra. The signs of an underactive throat chakra include introversion. While most people are likely to be an introvert than an extrovert depending on their personality traits, when the throat chakra is disrupted we tend to cut social connections out of our lives. This is because we become incapable of flawless communication and expressing our thoughts. The relationships that were built over a foundation of healthy communication fall because our mind shuts down. If left untreated this symptom can lead to total social isolation and existential crisis due to no human contact.

Another emotional side effect of an unbalanced throat chakra is the feeling of insecurity. Because we are unable to talk to other people, we often get consumed by our irrational thoughts. The usual drill is to communicate these insecurities to eliminate them from our mind. However, due to a blockage we tend to keep these insecurities to ourselves and it takes a toll on our self-esteem as well.

While these are the signs of a blocked throat chakra, the opposite happens when this chakra experiences over activity. Those individuals with an overactive throat chakra tend to lack control over their tongue and talk too much. They also lack the ability to filter their thoughts out before speaking. As the throat chakra becomes overwhelmed with energy, individuals can also be over-critical of themselves. They tend to attack their own thoughts, behaviors and emotions and as a result their relationships suffer as well. Additionally, those with a blocked chakra are very timid but individuals with an overactive throat chakra can often appear to be rude in their social settings. These individuals lack the regard for accepting ideas and concerns coming from other people and instead they exert their opinions.

THROAT CHAKRA MEDITATION TECHNIQUES

The symptoms of an imbalanced throat chakra must have alerted you by now. Are you wondering how you can balance your throat chakra? Restoring the balance and harmony in flow of energy through our body is essential for leading a calm and peaceful life. However, if there is a constant fluctuation in our chakra system it can keep us away from experiencing life in its fullest form. Nevertheless, there are several practices that can unclog the throat chakra. To begin with chakra healing techniques, you should make some behavioral changes as well:

1. **Using your voice:** As the throat chakra is the center of your voice it is important to practice speaking so that balance is restored. Although, you should not exert pressure on yourself to speak. Take your time and challenge yourself. Talking with close family members and friends can help you get out of this rut. As you try to speak your mind, it can eliminate the rustiness of your throat chakra and make it healthy again.
2. **Go outside:** None of the chakras can be healed if you are not allowing yourself some quiet and peaceful time. While throughout the week you are most likely to be busy, the weekend is when you put a stop to your work life. Spare some time for yourself to go outside and connect with nature. Sometimes all you need is a connection with mother Earth to feel grounded and secure.
3. **Physical activity:** Just like exercise is good for your body, it is also good for your chakra

system. Practicing yoga routinely can restore the energy in your throat chakra. There are several poses that are recommended by chakra scholars. The list of yoga positions for the benefit of your throat energy house includes[63]:

- Bridge pose
- Child's pose
- Upward plank pose
- Plow pose

While these techniques will put your mind at ease they will also help you strengthen your cognitive skills for meditation techniques:

1. **Throat chakra meditation:** A lifestyle change that chakra scholars always recommend is practicing meditation routinely for the good of your chakra system. Sit down with your shoulders back and keep your spine straight. Relax your tense muscles and take deep breaths to quiet down your mind. After that, build concentration on the location of the throat chakra. Once you can feel the sensation of your chakra, imagine a blue glowing light that is fueled by warmth. End the session when you unlock tranquility.

2. **Throat chakra affirmations:** Repeating positive affirmations is an interesting way of curing the negative effects of a blocked throat chakra. Some of the suggested affirmations that you can use during meditation include:

   - 'I should allow myself to speak nothing but the truth.'
   - 'I am capable of having an open and honest communication with others.'
   - 'I have the power to nourish my creative skills and self-expression.'
   - 'I know when to stop talking and listen.'
   - 'I have the desire to live an honest and authentic life.'
   - 'Communication will help me build healthy relationships.'

3. **Throat chakra crystal healing:** Each chakra can be aligned with the help of unique stones that radiate universal energy. When it comes to the throat chakra, the best gemstone is lapis lazuli. The common characteristic between the throat chakra and lapis lazuli is the color blue. Because of this tone, lapis lazuli syncs with our chakra and restores the balance. You can wear this stone as jewelry to take it with you on the go. You can also practice throat chakra meditation by placing this stone on the location of this energy vortex. Other crystals for throat

chakra include aquamarine, angelite, turquoise and blue kyanite[64].

MEDITATION GUIDE FOR THROAT CHAKRA

Are you having trouble sharing what you feel with your loved one? Is it taking away the excitement and life out of your relationship? Since you know what the symptoms of an imbalanced throat chakra is, it is time to make the smart decision and heal the damage that has been done to your energy house.

Meditation helps you resurrect your spirit. If you are falling apart that is because you have lost touch with your real self. We previously mentioned meditating with a throat chakra crystal. Now we will pick up from there and give you a beginner's guide to heal your throat chakra.

Before we start with the meditation practice for throat chakra, you will need to make a small investment in a throat chakra crystal. Lapis lazuli should be your first pick. However, if purchasing this blue stone is a little heavy on your wallet you can choose a cheaper option such as turquoise. These stones do not need to be refined and you can buy an uncut gem to save some money. If you can purchase several of your chosen blue stones it will help you generate more energy and heal your throat chakra fast.

Balance Your Chakras

Bring your new best friend home; we mean the gemstone that you have chosen! In your house, you should locate a place that makes you feel warm and secure. We all have our favorite spouts where we feel cozy and nice.

It is time to revamp this space. Start by placing your crystals around your chosen space because you will be meditating here quite often. Although, set aside one stone for later. Now that you are satisfied with your new interior decor. It is time to heal.

Take a nice hot shower to practice the relaxation that is required for crystal meditation. During this time you can indulge in some shower thoughts so that later your mind is clear.

Once you are done, make sure you put on some comfortable and easy clothes.

Now come back to your favorite spot and pick up that blue gemstone that you set aside. Lay down on the floor and place this stone on the location of your throat chakra. Once you are set you should close your eyes.

Take five deep breaths and focus on the rise and fall of your chest to relax yourself.

Once you are relaxed, you will focus on the weight of this crystal. This focus will help you become aware of the crystal and eventually you will feel it radiating through your chakra.

Lay down in that position for at least 10 minutes to let the crystal do its job. For this meditation, you do not need to put in extra effort. The powerful crystal will rewire your chakra. You just need to keep your mind at ease.

Once you feel calm, take a deep breath and open your eyes. Pick up the chakra crystal before you get off the floor. Finish the meditation and go about your day.

CHAPTER 9

The Third Eye Chakra

In this book we are taking off the veil from hidden knowledge about the various dimensions of our body. By now, we have established that our bodies are powered through the energy that flows in the universe. This is what gives us our sense of purpose and a connection with Earth. The only requirement for understanding human life through lenses other than hard science is open-mindedness. The more we know about the chakras, the more we can understand ourselves.

Knowing how your body is connected with everything will help you build meaningful relations in life. Now it's time to move towards the sixth energy house in our body. In this chapter, we reveal the wonder that is the third eye chakra. You will be analyzing your sixth chakra and learning how you can open it with minor changes in your lifestyle. Once you get an idea about what a healthy third eye chakra looks like, you will definitely want to indulge in self-healing!

WHAT MAKES THE THIRD EYE CHAKRA IMPORTANT?

The third eye chakra has various names in different cultures. This gives us an idea about how deeply embedded this ancient practice of opening the chakra system is. Also known as the brow chakra, in Sanskrit it is noted by three common names; *Ajna chakra, dvidak padma,* and *bhru madhya*. All of these terms loosely translate to 'command' and 'perception'. Through this it can be assumed that the sixth chakra is linked to the supreme element which is intellect.

According to yogic metaphysics, the *Ajna* chakra is a channel where we transcend duality. This duality is personal to us. It is the 'I' and the 'We' personalities. The 'I' personality is what separates us from other individuals and makes us unique whereas the 'We' personality is the identity we take on when we are involved in our community. Based on that, the most common color that represents the third eye chakra is purple when it is balanced and blue-purple when the energy is high in this vortex. Scholars often mention that this chakra is characterized further by its quality of smooth radiance that reminds individuals of the moon light.

Across scholarly texts, the location for the third eye chakra is between our eyebrows. Slightly above the nose bridge, this chakra is often confused to be found at the middle of our forehead. However, this misunderstanding has been corrected by chakra experts over the years. Because of its specific location, this chakra has a biological duty as well. It is mainly concerned with our pineal gland which has many characteristics; this gland regulates biorhythms, sleep cycle, attention, and perception. It gives us our consciousness and creates visual stimulations for us. The *Ajna* chakra needs to be balanced so that no hindrance is caused for these biological processes of our body.

With that, there are various behavioral and emotional effects of a functional third eye chakra. Through the sixth chakra we are able to understand our reality. It goes beyond our typical physical senses into the realm of energies[65]. This means that 'third eye chakra' is another name for our sixth sense; intuitive sensibility. For example, in terms of our relationships the sixth chakra helps us look beyond the vessel that is our body and connect with the soul of another person instead. Such a mystical capability helps us build long-lasting relationships that are free from worldly interference.

Those who are able to get in touch with their brow chakra also unlock mystical powers that humans have been rumored to possess. The third eye chakra can produce visions in our minds that are hard to describe verbally. These visions are an example of mastering clairvoyance and clairaudience. Do you ever feel like you need to escape a situation but you cannot put your finger on what is alerting you? That is clairvoyance. You are able to connect with your wisdom and the insight it provides you helps you survive and know things before they happen. This is why numerous individuals have had a keen interest in the third eye chakra.

As individuals are able to look at the world differently, the sixth chakra fuels their inspiration and creativity. You must have heard people sharing what their dreams showed them to do. This is actually their third eye chakra that is rewiring their brain and fueling their consciousness with new ideas, perspectives, and creations. Those who have an open sixth chakra are artistic and love to explore their life. They understand that the world is not just what is taught to us. They connect with their highest form and live a sublime life.

What are the symptoms of an unbalanced third eye chakra?

There is a power within each individual that has the capability to change the way we look at the world. This power is part of us in the form of the third eye chakra. In its healthy state, the sixth chakra enables us to see things in an abstract form. However, slightest imbalance in the third eye chakra can create havoc for our emotional, physical, and psychological well-being. This chakra plays a key role in limiting the negative experiences we are exposed to in our life. However, when this portal to our sixth sense is blocked, our mind and body suffer through various side-effects.

The first thing that happens when the third eye chakra is blocked is losing the sense of direction of life. In other words, our intuition becomes rusty and our judgement becomes clouded. Even in small-scale everyday life situations, we are unable to make decisions and we feel lost when we are asked to navigate through these events. The idea we have in our head about life and our path becomes blurred. What once drove us with passion becomes stagnant in life. As a side-effect of this confused consciousness we also start to distrust our inner voice. The gut feeling we get when we are in a threatening situation becomes the cause of our paranoia leading us to block it out of our heads.

Through our sixth sense we are able to get closure and know where our life is headed but when this is removed from our bodies we become fearful of the future[66]. The beliefs, routine, and schemas we have in our mind before our third eye chakra becomes imbalanced start to shatter and become weak. Our consciousness becomes overwhelmed with irrational fears and we tend to develop existential crises which further takes a toll on our mental health.

As these symptoms consume our mind, body and soul we also lose the zest for life and motivation to meet our targets. From time to time, procrastination is welcomed. It helps us relax before we take the next big step in our life. However, when the third eye chakra is blocked we lose touch with our motivation and become lazy. If affected individuals are left in this state for too long, they can develop a distorted sense of reality.

People with a blocked third eye chakra fail to perceive the world beyond its physical manifestation. That means that they become consumed with materialistic thoughts and actions. The world as we know it requires intellect more than wealth to be dissected and understood. It is our purpose to unlock the wonders of nature. However, with an imbalanced sixth chakra individuals become less clairvoyant and slowly the other chakras in our body also start to suffer.

As the third eye chakra is linked to the pineal gland, there are various physical downsides of an imbalanced *Ajna* chakra as well. When this chakra becomes congested the various physical changes include dizziness, headaches and weak brain structure[67]. The gland that is responsible for our vision also starts to suffer and we experience hormonal imbalance as well. As a result, our vision can get affected. You might notice that your vision that used to be sharp once is now rusty. Long-term blockage in the sixth chakra might even push you to get visual aid. Due to this hormonal imbalance, individuals also develop extreme anxiety and depression. Some people even report losing their desire to go outside their houses.

HOW TO OPEN YOUR THIRD EYE CHAKRA AT HOME

Wouldn't you feel better if you didn't experience an emotional rollercoaster each day without a known cause? The downfalls of blocked third eye chakra can make even the tiniest life experience an anxiety explosion. In that case, there are various types of techniques especially designed to open the sixth chakra. Unlike the complex nature of this energy channel, these therapeutic remedies are simple. The following are some of the changes you must make in your behavior before we move towards the recommended treatments for third eye chakra:

- **Third eye chakra diet suggestions:** As intuitive as the *Ajna* chakra is, it requires a boost each day to function smoothly. There are various fruits and vegetables that you can purchase and stock in order to promote the opening of your sixth chakra. These include dark chocolate which provides you with mental clarity and concentration. Purple teas, fruits, and vegetables radiate the same energy as this chakra and making them part of your diet will restore the balance in this vortex. Lastly, eat some Omega-3 rich foods to boost your cognitive functions and protect your vision.

- **Embrace nature:** One of the biggest hurdles we face because of congested third eye chakra is consumption by materialistic items. If you have made up your mind to get your life together, connect with the nature around you from time to time. Forget sitting in front of the television and loathing your life. Instead of that, go outside and talk a nice long walk in the park. If you have access to a beach, now is the perfect time to sit by the shore and take in the view. This will help you understand that you are part of Earth and its wonders.

Once you have captured the necessity of making these behavioral changes, it is time to make some lifestyle changes and practice the following techniques to open your third eye chakra:

1. **Third eye chakra affirmations:** These are phrases that you repeat to yourself in order to target limiting and negative beliefs that are confusing your mind due to blockage of the third eye chakra. As you repeat them to yourself, they can slowly replace previous rusty beliefs with more positive beliefs. Affirmations for the brow chakra focus on gut instincts, spirituality, and sense of purpose. The following are some of the best phrases you can use while you are meditating or on your lunch break:

    - 'I follow the lead of my intuition.'
    - 'I have the ability to make the right decisions with ease.'

- 'I can hear my intuitions and they will bring me closer to my purpose.'
- 'I am on the right path.'
- 'I am able to see the world by connecting to its spiritual realm.'

2. **Third eye chakra stone meditation and jewelry:** The purpose behind assigning each chakra its color is to help you find tools in nature that correspond to its energy because they share the same tones. Using this information, you can locate various gemstones that resonate the *Ajna* chakra. You can carry these stones on you in your bag or accessorize your outfit instead. When you meditate you can also place these gemstones on the location of your third eye chakra to restart the power. Some of the best recommended stones for this energy hub are amethyst, black obsidian, and purple fluorite. You can even make a combination of various purple stones to reincarnate your sixth chakra at a faster pace. The best thing about this remedy is that these stones require the least amount of investment[68].

Third Eye Chakra Guided Meditation

Each chakra needs to be in tune with other chakras to make sure we connect to our emotional, physical, and spiritual qualities. For thousands of years, aromatherapy has been used to soothe the mind and soul. As a result, these essential oils rewire our body and we are able to get back on track. For chakra healing, essential oil is one of the cheapest solutions that can help you reconnect with your third eye chakra. Each energy house is assigned an essential oil depending on their characteristics and aura. In the case of the third eye chakra, we will recommend you to use rosemary essential oil.

Before you make the purchase, you should understand why rosemary works well with the third eye chakra. When your sixth chakra is combined with the essence of rosemary, it awakens your third eye and reshapes your perception and concentration. Similar to that, there are some other oils that you can purchase in case rosemary has an aversive effect on you. These include sandalwood, chamomile, and frankincense[69].

The first step of this guided meditation is going to the market and picking out one of these scents. Take your time and test them out because you will be using these essential oils for a longer period to awaken your third eye chakra. Once you have made the suitable choice, we can move forward with the meditation.

There are two things you need to do before you go into the meditation pose. Firstly, to practice aromatherapy you will put a couple of drops of the multi-purpose essential oil in an incense burner. While you do this, make sure to take safety precautions. After you are done, let the aroma fill the room and dim the lights as well.

The second thing you need to do before meditation is rub the oil on your forehead. Take a few drops and rub the area associated with the third eye chakra. This will help warm up the chakra and intensify the meditation process.

Now that you have done both of these things, you have taken care of most of the work. In this room now, you will be choosing a space where you feel the most comfortable. Make sure to remove any irritating jewelry, makeup and change into cozy clothes to relax yourself without any outwardly interruption.

Once you have found your spot, place a yoga mat on the floor and lie down. You will keep an upright position with your arms on the side and your legs straight. After that, you will close your eyes and take five deep breaths.

As you concentrate on your breath you will go into a deep relaxation state. This is essential to make sure that your third eye chakra therapy is working in its favor.

After you are relaxed, imagine that you are enveloped in a purple energy that is coming out of your third eye chakra. Keep imagining this state and take deep breaths from time to time.

Your job is just to keep a calm mind here. Once you are done with your session and you can go back to your routine. Repeat this meditation several times a week to avail its benefits.

CHAPTER 10

The Crown Chakra

The philosophy behind the chakra system helps us understand that the universe has many gifts through which humans can find enlightenment in life. What makes us whole and boosts our confidence is not the material we can possess. It is connecting with the universe around us that gives us our purpose in life and fulfills us. Keeping this in mind, opening your chakras is not just about self-healing. Even those who are healthy are encouraged to practice chakra meditation because it brings us back in touch with the Divine.

Moving forward with the chakra system, we are going to discuss the seventh and last chakra in our body; the crown chakra. Just like the root chakra, this channel must be balanced at all times so that energy can pass through the whole system without interruption. You will get the gist of what a crown chakra can do for you when it is open. With that, we will share symptoms of an unhealthy seventh chakra and finish it through a complete healing guide.

How an Open Crown Chakra Functions

The color of your crown chakra is violet. This tone has been allotted to the last chakra because it signifies your connection with energies coming from heaven. As violet is a spiritual color, it has the strongest vibration of all the colors in the light spectrum. This color also gives us a sense of oneness and wholeness while keeping our mind at peace. Violet is also a promise of something new coming in your life. This shade signifies spiritual illumination and rebirth. Through the crown chakra we are able to let go of sadness and inner conflicts and transcend in life. Lastly, the color violet is purifying for the soul, mind, and body. It brings us in touch with realities that exist beyond our material reality.

The seven chakra can be found at the top of our heads. Primarily, the crown chakra is linked with the pituitary gland, the hypothalamus, and the pineal gland. This chakra makes sure that these glands are working together to regulate our endocrine growth and strengthen our body. Additionally, the location of crown chakra also gives it access to our brain and the nervous system. These are two major parts of our body and they are supervised by the crown chakra to make sure they remain protected.

Chakra scholars associate the crown chakra with our consciousness and intuitive knowledge as well. While the third eye chakra helps us see multiple realities, the crown chakra is responsible for taking that information and creating an awareness of our higher consciousness. When the crown chakra is unlocked, we get access to the ultimate connection with our spirituality. In the chakra system, this energy house represents our independence from the mortal world. Instead, we are able to shift our focus on the divine planes and our psychic gifts.

When your crown chakra is activated you begin to let go of any perceived limitations in your life. Instead of believing that you lack some qualities, the crown chakra helps you realize that the only person stopping you from achieving your dreams is you. Traditionally, the crown chakra is a portal to self-knowledge. Even in our thirties most of us are unable to know who we really are. We are consumed by insecurities that block us from accessing our true potential. However, the crown chakra is a channel of empowerment. It helps us see through ourselves and find answers to our problems from within[70].

In our world there are various hubs of false wisdom that astray us from our true path in life. These dualistic theories about the universe are designed to confuse us and alienate us from seeing beyond the physical world. Although, with the help of your crown chakra you are able to separate the truth from false knowledge. It sharpens your mind to find clarity in life.

The crown chakra symbol is made with a lotus flower in violet tone. This flower has thousand petals in total and each one signifies renewal, purity, and beauty of the human soul. Some individuals choose to get the crown chakra symbol tattooed on their body to remember its existence and resonate their seventh chakra.

The crown chakra is the reason behind our mystical experiences with other beings in the universe. With that, the crown chakra is also responsible for what is popularly categorized as the 'deja-vu' experience. Many of us have had experienced moments in our life that make us suspect that the past has repeated itself. The feeling that 'this has already happened before' is the ability of the crown chakra to connect us with our past, present, and future[71].

SIGNS YOUR CROWN CHAKRA IS IMBALANCED

Now that you have an idea about a functional crown chakra, you might be wondering how you can know when your seventh chakra is blocked. Understanding why the crown chakra blocks is important so that when you attempt to heal your chakra the therapies are effective. Your crown chakra can experience congestion because of emotionally upsetting life experiences such as loss, conflict, and/or traumatic incidents. Losing someone close to you can slow you down and consume you with sadness. Your mind replays old memories and many of us become prone to staying stuck in that moment. While your emotions can make your crown chakra rusty, it is your psychological state that can block you from connecting with your higher self. Those who constantly experience stress, fear, and anxiety begin to experience malfunctioning of the crown chakra. When these blockages are not treated they can result in psychological and emotional disorders.

People with an overactive crown chakra tend to become pompous and lofty. In other words, such individuals are driven to stick by their rigid beliefs and lack open-mindedness. With a very dogmatic personality, they are also at the risk of becoming disconnected with their reality. Instead of believing that you are just like everyone else, you can become narcissistic. An overactive crown chakra leads you to obtaining other negative personality characteristics such as obsessiveness, greed, selfishness, and secretive nature. Such individuals are also hypocritical and fail to make people place their trust in them. Such characteristics can be very threatening to the health of your personal and professional relationships in life. As partners, individuals with overactive seventh chakra are extremely controlling and critical of their loved ones. In their professional life, they are incredibly dismissive of others around them and fail to work in a group setting[72].

People with overactive crown chakra are often consumed with feeling disoriented and lost in life. Some individuals have to battle depression while others become destructive eventually. While people with a healthy crown chakra view life with passion, an imbalanced seventh chakra can make us feel distant. As the constant frustration irritates you, it becomes hard for you to realize the power you hold within and you experience difficulty in learning. There are various physical symptoms that occur when there is an imbalance in your crown chakra. These include sudden light sensitivity, dissociation, dizziness, and cognitive impairments.

Life loses its meaning when the crown chakra is blocked. What used to motivate you each morning does not make sense anymore. Through our personal connections, we are able to feel whole. However, the relations that used to excite you become experiences of loneliness. When your crown chakra is congested, it can be hard to understand why humans were placed on Earth. The divine knowledge that used to bring you peace stops making sense when you are unable to access your crown chakra completely. In such a state, individuals become materialistic and hoard possessions instead of finding their purpose in life.

This lack of belief in the Divine also makes us prone to making negative choices in life. Every action we make has a consequence. We all are capable of having destructive thoughts but the crown chakra acts as a filter and helps us make the right choice after weighing the negative and positive consequences of a decision we are about to take. This helps us protect ourselves from making poor choices that can hurt us and others around us. Although when your crown chakra is not functioning at its optimal level you fail to think your actions through often making decisions that have side effects[73].

How to heal your crown chakra

You must be feeling out of sorts because your crown chakra is not aligned with your mind and body. Feeling detached from the world stops us from progressing in life which is why it is important to cleanse and heal your crown chakra. Once you have self-analyzed and noted down any emotional, physical and psychological imbalances, you will be even more motivated to open your crown chakra. Beware that if you leave your crown chakra congested for a longer time it can lead to various physical challenges such as epilepsy, cancer, headaches, brain tumors, amnesia, and pituitary problems. Following are several steps you can take to reconnect with your crown chakra and restore your gifts:

- **Crown chakra meditation:** While it is hard to alter your lifestyle you must push yourself in order to influence your crown chakra positively. Introduce meditation to your daily schedule. That is because only through a peaceful mind you will be able to connect with higher energies in the universe that will in turn balance your crown chakra. Even if you have a few minutes to meditate, sit down in a comfortable position and imagine a violet ray at the top of your head. Through imagining this you will stimulate your seventh chakra and open it eventually.

- **Forget your ego:** Having confidence in yourself and being driven by your ego are two separate experiences. Self-confidence helps you push your ideas forward without dismissing others whereas ego makes you look down on people. In order to let your crown chakra bloom you must release yourself from your ego. To do that, you should process your insecurities because that is what fuels ego.

- **Practice 'seva':** *'Seva'* is a Sanskrit word for serving other people around you. It means helping those in need and indulging in some community work. By taking care of other people you realize that there is power in unity. Through other humans, you are able to gain knowledge that you have lost. So in order to rewire your crown chakra, you just need to be kind to others.

- **Unconditionally love yourself and others:** Due to the side-effects of a blocked crown chakra it must be hard for you to choose love over negative thoughts and actions. However, just like humans are inherently destructive they are also capable of love. In that case, you must stop yourself from making quick and unthoughtful decisions and take a moment to choose love when you are around others. This also includes finding things you love about yourself and focusing on them instead of being overly critical of yourself.

- **Aromatherapy:** Another step that you can take to open your crown chakra is very light on your wallet. You can go to your local market and purchase some recommended essential oils for your crown chakra. These include lavender, jasmine and rose. The wild range of scents that you can use for aromatherapy bring you tranquility which helps your crown chakra connect with the energy coming from dimensions around you[74].

- **Pump up your wardrobe:** While opening your chakra you can also have some fun. Chakra healers believe that wearing clothing items that are purple can open your crown chakra. That is because purple and violet tones of your clothes are able to produce vibrations at a frequency that can restore balance in your seventh chakra. In addition to that, you can also invest in healing crystals and wear them as necklaces. Natural crystals that help unclog the crown chakra include clear quartz, selenite, and amethyst. In case you have a budget, you can wear diamonds to help your crown chakra open up[75].

Meditation guide for crown chakra

Would you like to regain your intuitive knowledge and deep understanding of what the universe is hiding behind the physical realm? The following meditation script will use your power of imagination to open your eyes and help you use your crown chakra to the fullest:

In order to start, you should sit in a comfortable meditation position. The traditional way to do this is by sitting with your legs crossed while keeping your back straight.

Place your hands in your lap. Make sure that you keep your palms upward. Now put your left hand on top of your right hand. This is called *'mudra'* and through this hand position you will be able to receive energy.

Now you must close your eyes and take slow and even breaths.

Calm down as you breathe.

Moving on, you will visualize a lotus with thousand petals located at the top of your head. Imagine that the petals are gently opening to unleash a violet light that the lotus holds. This is a virtual image of your crown chakra.

Continue to imagine the lotus on your head. Through your sense of imagination you are letting the divine light of this universe flow down into your body through the crown chakra. Now that you have a strong visualization of the chakra, you will participate in repeating the following chakra affirmations to yourself:

'I am surrounded by the protective divine light.'
'This violet light will nourish my entire being.'
'I am forever walking in the violet light.'
'I grow stronger by following the divine light.'

After repeating these affirmations several times, you can move forward to the next step when you feel ready.

Now you will imagine this purple light coming out of the lotus. This ray of light is spiraling down your spine and with it comes a warmth that brings your body alive. Your imagination is no longer a picture in your head but it is a portal of energy through which your consciousness will soon be illuminated.

In the next step, you will focus all of your senses on how intense the light is. As you concentrate without interruption, you will be able to taste, smell, hear, and touch this violet light. This is a manifestation of your higher self.

In your mind, you have reached the Divine and you are holding this position to let it resurrect your crown chakra. You will be holding this position for another 15 minutes.

Now it's time for you to come out of this meditation. Slowly open your eyes and with it take deep and even breaths. Now that your eyes are opened repeat the previous affirmations to yourself. The more you repeat the more you will believe in them.

Because this is an intense meditation, it requires practice and repetition. If you cannot get it right in the first try, don't be frustrated. With time you will be able to sharpen your imagination and concentration. As you do that, your crown chakra will bloom too.

Final Thoughts

All chakras in our body are aligned with our spine from top to bottom. With that, these chakras make their presence known when they regulate the glands in our body. These energy channels are responsible for making our body function smoothly while keeping our mind at ease. Each chakra has a different rotational speed and frequency of the energy it radiates. When they are combined together, they ensure physical and psychological health. The chakra system also communicates with you when it is healthy and when it needs your rescue. The key is to listen to your body. Depression, stress, and anxiety are common non-verbal signs that are used by the chakra system to alert you of underlying imbalances.

The upper chakras are concerned with spirituality whereas lower chakras in your body are concerned with meeting your basic needs of food, shelter, and love. Together these chakras are your inner powerhouse that give you your personality, sense of reality, perception, and goal in life. In order to make sure you move forward in life, you should also observe your body. As each chakra is located in a specific place, it affects the organs located around the spot. Any disorders of such organs is a sign that you must take a step back in life and heal.

The chakra system is a prehistoric discovery but we can notice that modern science is slowly warming up to the theories behind it. Empirical science can only bring you explanations for some aspects of the universe but with the chakra system you can open up the mysteries of the universe through your body. There are various life experiences in our mind for which we are unable to find an explanation using modern medicine. However, what lacks in objective science is covered by alternate medicine and knowing the chakra system is essential for healing yourself.

After covering the specifics of the crown chakra we have come to an end. Although, for disciples of the chakra system this end is a beginning of their self-healing journey. Consuming intrinsic details about the seven chakras; root chakra, sacral chakra, solar plexus chakra, heart chakra, throat chakra, third eye chakra, and crown chakra gives you an idea of what your life will become once you stop chasing the material world. Ancient scholars passed down the knowledge of the chakra system to each generation because it is essential for human beings to never forget their roots.

Each meditation guide has been designed to give beginners a hand when they start with chakra healing. These meditation techniques require a little practice, which is why staying patient is mandatory to open all of your chakras. The chakra system is a lifestyle change. It requires you to leave behind your understanding of the physical world and how your body works. Anything that you have learnt in the past is no longer the explanation you will look for when understanding your surroundings. Instead of that, opening your chakras will help you get in touch with higher wisdom that is held by the universe for thousands of years.

Endnotes

1. Conventry, Anna. "An Introduction To The Chakras". *DOYOU.COM*, 2020, https://www.doyou.com/an-introduction-to-the-chakras-for-beginners-36252/.
2. "Chakra". *En.Wikipedia.Org*, 2020, https://en.wikipedia.org/wiki/Chakra.
3. Graybill et al., John. *The Chakra Journey*. 1st ed., Lulu, 2013, pp. 8-9, Accessed 1 Apr 2020.
4. "3 Simple Steps To Open Your Chakras". *Chakras.Info*, 2019, https://www.chakras.info/opening-chakras/.
5. "Elements Of The Seven Chakras". *Energyenhancement.Org*, 2020, http://www.energyenhancement.org/chakras/Chakra_general/elements%20of%20chakras.html#three.
6. "Elements Of The Seven Chakras". *Energyenhancement.Org*, 2020, http://www.energyenhancement.org/chakras/Chakra_general/elements%20of%20chakras.html#three.
7. Studies, Tantrik. "The Real Story On The Chakras — Tantrik Studies". *Tantrik Studies*, 2020, https://hareesh.org/blog/2016/2/5/the-real-story-on-the-chakras.
8. "Elements Of The Seven Chakras". *Energyenhancement.Org*, 2020, http://www.energyenhancement.org/chakras/Chakra_general/elements%20of%20chakras.html#three.
9. "A Guide To The Seven Chakras And Their Meanings". *One Tribe Apparel*, 2020, https://www.onetribeapparel.com/blogs/pai/seven-chakras-meaning.
10. "The 7 Chakras". *Deities*, 2020, https://deitiesstore.com/blogs/news/the-7-chakras.
11. "Hindu Gods And Goddesses". *Thehindugods.Com*, 2020, https://www.thehindugods.com/.

12. Polizzi, Nick. "The Ancient Art Of Chakra Bathing - The Sacred Science". *The Sacred Science*, 2020, https://www.thesacredscience.com/the-ancient-art-of-chakra-bathing/.
13. "The Real Truth About The Chakras". *UPLIFT*, 2020, https://upliftconnect.com/truth-about-the-chakras/.
14. Studies, Tantrik. "The Real Story On The Chakras — Tantrik Studies". *Tantrik Studies*, 2020, https://hareesh.org/blog/2016/2/5/the-real-story-on-the-chakras.
15. Binford, Harry. "The Rainbow Body: How The Western Chakra System Came To Be". *Theosophical.Org*, 2020, https://www.theosophical.org/publications/quest-magazine/4246-the-rainbow-body-how-the-western-chakra-system-came-to-be.
16. Marshall, Michael. "The Secret Of How Life On Earth Began". *Bbc.Com*, 2020, http://www.bbc.com/earth/story/20161026-the-secret-of-how-life-on-earth-began.
17. "Benjamin Moore (Biochemist) - Biotic Energy". *Liquisearch.Com*, 2020, https://www.liquisearch.com/benjamin_moore_biochemist/biotic_energy.
18. "Plato'S View On The Souls". *Ukessays.Com*, 2020, https://www.ukessays.com/essays/philosophy/platos-view-on-the-souls-philosophy-essay.php.
19. "Six Pillars Of Energy Medicine - Energy Medicine With Donna Eden - Energy Medicine With Donna Eden". *Innersource.Net*, 2020, https://www.innersource.net/em/107-resources/publishedarticles/283-sixpillarsofem.html.
20. "Six Pillars Of Energy Medicine - Energy Medicine With Donna Eden - Energy Medicine With Donna Eden". *Innersource.Net*, 2020, https://www.innersource.net/em/107-resources/publishedarticles/283-sixpillarsofem.html.
21. Writer, Elizabeth. "What Is Reiki?". *Livescience.Com*, 2020, https://www.livescience.com/40275-reiki.html.
22. "The Science Behind CHAKRAS - Powerthoughts Meditation Club". *Powerthoughts Meditation Club*, 2020, http://powerthoughtsmeditationclub.com/the-chakras/.

23 Orzel, Chad. "Six Things Everyone Should Know About Quantum Physics". *Forbes*, 2020, https://www.forbes.com/sites/chadorzel/2015/07/08/six-things-everyone-should-know-about-quantum-physics/#9fe80007d467.

24 Tabish, Syed. "Complementary And Alternative Healthcare: Is It Evidence-Based?". *Pubmed Central (PMC)*, 2020, https://www.ncbi.nlm.nih.gov/pmc/articles/PMC3068720/.

25 "Ancient Indian Healing Part 2: Practices For Physical, Mental And Emotional Well-Being". *The Mindful Word*, 2020, https://www.themindfulword.org/2016/ancient-indian-energy-healing-practices.

26 Warber, Sara L et al. "A Consideration of the Perspectives of Healing Practitioners on Research Into Energy Healing." *Global advances in health and medicine* vol. 4,Suppl (2015): 72-8. doi:10.7453/gahmj.2015.014.suppl

27 Ross, Christina L. "Energy Medicine: Current Status and Future Perspectives." *Global advances in health and medicine* vol. 8 2164956119831221. 27 Feb. 2019, doi:10.1177/2164956119831221

28 Maxwell, Richard. (2009). The Physiological Foundation of Yoga Chakra Expression. Zygon®. 44. 807 - 824. 10.1111/j.1467-9744.2009.01035.x.

29 Cogan, Shannon. "Chakras: The Psychology Of Extraordinary Beliefs". *U.Osu.Edu*, 2020, https://u.osu.edu/vanzandt/2018/04/18/chakras/.

30 "Yoga's Energy Centers: What Science Says About The Chakras". *Yogauonline.Com*, 2020, https://yogauonline.com/yoga-research/yogas-energy-centers-what-science-says-about-chakras.

31 Judith, Anodea. Eastern Body, Western Mind: Psychology and the Chakra System As a Path to the Self. Berkeley, Calif: Celestial Arts, 2004.

32 Meriwether, Nana. "Is There Scientific Proof For The Existence Of Chakras? A Brief Introduction To Chakras And The

Compelling Science Behind The Energy Found Within Us All". *Welltheresthis.Com*, 2020, https://www.welltheresthis.com/single-post/2018/07/05/Week-27-Is-There-Scientific-Proof-for-the-Existence-of-Chakras-A-Brief-Introduction-to-Chakras-and-The-Compelling-Science-Behind-The-Energy-Found--Within-Us-All.

33 Wisneski, Len, and Lucy Anderson. "The scientific basis of integrative medicine." (2005): 257-259.

34 Wisneski, Len, and Lucy Anderson. "The Scientific Basis of Integrative Medicine." *Evidence-based Complementary and Alternative Medicine* vol. 2,2 (2005): 257–259. doi:10.1093/ecam/neh079

35 "The Science Of Chakras". *Mind Bender*, 2020, https://mind-bender.co/the-science-of-chakras/.

36 Gronich, Ari. "Is There Scientific Evidence For Chakras?". *Achieve Health USA*, 2020, https://achievehealthusa.com/is-there-scientific-evidence-for-chakras/.

37 Freshwater, Shawna. "1St Chakra Root Muladhara". *Shawna Freshwater, Phd*, 2020, https://spacioustherapy.com/1st-chakra-root-muladhara/.

38 "7 Facts About The Root Chakra You Should Know". *Astrologyanswers.Com*, 2020, https://astrologyanswers.com/article/root-chakra-facts-healing/.

39 "Alchemy Of Stability: Earth Energy Of Root Chakra". *DOYOU.COM*, 2020, https://www.doyou.com/alchemy-of-stability-earth-energy-of-root-chakra-48245/.

40 "The Root Chakra: Muladhara". *The Chopra Center*, 2020, https://chopra.com/articles/the-root-chakra-muladhara.

41 Robinson, Aspen. "Root Chakra & Emotions". *Augustknoxnomad.Com*, 2020, https://augustknoxnomad.com/root-chakra-emotions/.

42 Shah, Parita. "9 Signs Your Root Chakra Energy Is Grounded". *Yogiapproved*™, 2020, https://www.yogiapproved.com/om/grounded-root-chakra/.

43 V., Andreea. "15 Signs Your Root Chakra Is Blocked And How To Heal It". *Learning Mind*, 2020, https://www.learning-mind.com/root-chakra-blocked/.

44 Luna, Aletheia. "The Ultimate Guide To Root Chakra Healing For Complete Beginners". *Lonerwolf*, 2020, https://lonerwolf.com/root-chakra-healing/.

45 "3 Easy Ways To Fix Root Chakra Imbalance". *Arhanta Yoga Ashram*, 2020, https://www.arhantayogaindia.com/muladhara-root-chakra-imbalance/.

46 "Muladhara: The Importance Of The Root Chakra And How To Open It". *Brainwavepowermusic.Com*, 2020, https://brainwavepowermusic.com/blog/blog/muladhara-the-importance-of-the-root-chakra-and-how-to-open-it.

47 "7 Facts You Should Know About The Sacral Chakra". *Astrologyanswers.Com*, 2020, https://astrologyanswers.com/article/sacral-chakra-facts-healing/.

48 Ness, Katie, and Katie Ness. "Sacral Chakra: Here'S Everything You Need To Know About Your Second Chakra". *Yogiapproved*, 2020, https://www.yogiapproved.com/om/the-second-chakra-how-it-impacts-your-relationships-and-creativity/.

49 Houston, Diana. "The Sacral Chakra: Meanings, Properties And Powers - A Complete Guide". *Crystalsandjewelry.Com*, 2020, https://meanings.crystalsandjewelry.com/sacral-chakra/.

50 Hurst, Katherine. "Sacral Chakra Healing For Beginners: How To Open Your Sacral Chakra". *The Law Of Attraction*, 2020, https://www.thelawofattraction.com/sacral-chakra-healing/.

51 Levin, Jordanna. "Foods That Balance Your Sacral Chakra". *Jordanna Levin*, 2020, https://jordannalevin.com/foods-that-balance-your-sacral-chakra/.

52 "Everything You Need To Know About The Solar Plexus Chakra". *Mindvalley Blog*, 2020, https://blog.mindvalley.com/solar-plexus-chakra/.

53 "Solar Plexus Chakra". *Chakras.Info*, 2020, https://www.chakras.info/solar-plexus-chakra/.

54 Hurst, Katherine. "Solar Plexus Chakra Healing: How To Open Your Solar Plexus Chakra". *The Law Of Attraction*, 2020, https://www.thelawofattraction.com/solar-plexus-chakra-healing/.

55 Howie, Vicki. "7 Ways To Fulfill The Need Of Your Solar Plexus Chakra". *Conscious Life News*, 2020, https://consciouslifenews.com/7-ways-fulfill-need-solar-plexus-chakra/1183404/#.

56 "The Heart Chakra". *Chakras.Info*, 2020, https://www.chakras.info/heart-chakra/.

57 Ness, Katie. "Heart Chakra: Here'S Everything You Need To Know About Your Fourth Chakra". *Yogiapproved™*, 2020, https://www.yogiapproved.com/om/the-heart-chakra-how-it-impacts-your-ability-to-love-and-be-loved/.

58 "11 Signs Your Heart Chakra Is Blocked & It's Messing With Your Love Life". *Bustle*, 2020, https://www.bustle.com/p/11-signs-your-heart-chakra-is-blocked-its-messing-with-your-love-life-8058873.

59 Luna, Aletheia. "The Ultimate Guide To Heart Chakra Healing For Complete Beginners". *Lonerwolf*, 2020, https://lonerwolf.com/heart-chakra-healing/.

60 "20 Powerful Heart Chakra Affirmations To Open Your Heart Space". *Through The Phases*, 2020, https://www.throughthephases.com/powerful-heart-chakra-affirmations/.

61 "Throat Chakra". *Chakra Anatomy*, 2020, https://www.chakra-anatomy.com/throat-chakra.html.

62 "Throat Chakra". *Chakras.Info*, 2020, https://www.chakras.info/throat-chakra/.

63 "Chakra Healing: How To Open Your Throat Chakra". *Goodnet*, 2020, https://www.goodnet.org/articles/chakra-healing-how-to-open-your-throat.

64 "5 Ways To Heal Your Throat Chakra". *Mindvalley Blog*, 2020, https://blog.mindvalley.com/throat-chakra-healing/.

65 "Third Eye Chakra". *Chakras.Info*, 2020, https://www.chakras.info/third-eye-chakra/.

66 "11 Signs That Your Third Eye Chakra Is Blocked, Imbalanced Or Underactive". *Spirilution.Com*, 2020, https://www.spirilution.com/blogs/featured-blog-posts/11-signs-that-your-third-eye-is-blocked-imbalanced-or-underactive.

67 "How To Tell If One Or More Of Your Chakras Are Blocked". *Third Eye Transcend*, 2020, https://thirdeyetranscend.com/blogs/mindfulness-blog/how-to-tell-if-one-or-more-of-your-chakras-are-blocked.

68 Hurst, Katherine. "Third Eye Chakra Healing For Beginners: How To Open Your Third Eye". *The Law Of Attraction*, 2020, https://www.thelawofattraction.com/third-eye-chakra-healing/.

69 "Using Essential Oils To Balance Each Of The 7 Chakras". *Auracacia.Com*, 2020, https://www.auracacia.com/community/article/using-essential-oils-to-balance-each-of-the-7-chakras.

70 "Crown Chakra - Sahasrara". *Chakra Anatomy*, 2020, https://www.chakra-anatomy.com/crown-chakra.html.

71 Houston, Diana. "The Crown Chakra: Meanings, Properties And Powers". *Crystalsandjewelry.Com*, 2020, https://meanings.crystalsandjewelry.com/crown-chakra/.

72 "5 Warning Signs Your Chakras Are Out Of Balance". *The Chopra Center*, 2020, https://chopra.com/articles/5-warning-signs-your-chakras-are-out-of-balance.

73 "Is Your Crown Chakra In Balance?". *Anna Sayce*, 2020, https://www.annasayce.com/is-your-crown-chakra-in-balance/.

74 "Chakra Healing: How To Open Your Crown Chakra". *Goodnet*, 2020, https://www.goodnet.org/articles/chakra-healing-how-to-open-your-crown.

75 "Crown Chakra Healing With Crystals". *Thehealingchest.Com*, 2020, https://thehealingchest.com/crystals-stones/crown-chakra-healing-with-crystals/.

Thank you for getting our book!

If you enjoy using it and you found it useful in your journey of spiritual growth and healing, we would greatly appreciate your review on Amazon.

Just head on over to this book's Amazon page and click "Write a customer review".

We read each and every one of them. Thanks!

www.ingramcontent.com/pod-product-compliance
Lightning Source LLC
Chambersburg PA
CBHW071717020426
42333CB00017B/2299